MACULAR DEGENERATION

and other

DISEASES OF THE AGING EYE

Diagnosis & Treatments

2014 Report

A Special Report
published in conjunction with
Cleveland Clinic's Cole Eye Institute

Macular Degeneration and other Diseases of the Aging Eye: Diagnosis & Treatments

Consulting Editor: Andrew P. Schachat, MD, Vice Chairman, Cole Eye Institute, Cleveland Clinic

Author: Karen Rafinski

Group Directors, Belvoir Media Group: Diane Muhlfeld, Jay Roland

Creative Director, Belvoir Media Group: Judi Crouse

Editor: Kristine Lang

Contributing Editor: David C. Holzman

Illustrations, images: Marty Bee, Thinkstock

Publisher, Belvoir Media Group: Timothy H. Cole

ISBN: 1-879620-81-2

To order additional copies of this report or for customer service questions, please call 877-300-0253, go to www.heart-advisor.com, or write to Health Special Reports, 800 Connecticut Avenue, Norwalk, CT 06854-1631.

2014

Macular Degeneration
and other Diseases of the Aging Eye
Diagnosis & Treatments

Age brings with it wisdom and experience, but it also brings an increased risk for illness—particularly of the eyes. In fact, most of the eye diseases that are to blame for reduced vision—including macular degeneration, glaucoma, and cataracts—are age-related. As an increasing percentage of the American population grows older, the threat of these diseases, and with them significant vision loss, increases. More than two-thirds of people with vision impairment are over age 65, according to the National Eye Institute.

This report was designed to be your guide to the changes that can affect your vision as you get older. It begins with many of the most common sight-robbing conditions—explaining what symptoms to look for, and what to do if you suspect you have an eye problem. Even more important, within these pages you'll learn critical prevention strategies that can help you preserve your vision and avoid many of these diseases before they have a chance to compromise your vision.

NEW FINDINGS

▶ Latest results show lutein, zeaxanthin help slow AMD; omega-3s do not
(Page 21, Box 2-5)

▶ Lucentis works better on wet AMD when combined with Fovista (Page 24, Box 2-7)

▶ Cataract surgery associated with reduced hip fractures (Page 40, Box 4-2)

▶ Anti-convulsant topiramate may raise glaucoma risk (Page 51, Box 5-3)

▶ Peripheral vision loss from glaucoma may increase auto crash risk
(Page 54, Box 5-4)

▶ Insertion of tiny drains may improve control of intraocular pressure
(Page 57, Box 5-5)

▶ Link between rise in diabetes and non-refractive visual impairment
(Page 63, Box 6-1)

▶ Lucentis approved for diabetic macular edema (Page 68, Box 6-3)

▶ Type 2 diabetes drug effective against diabetic retinopathy (Page 68, Box 6-4)

▶ Tablets boost speed and comfort for readers with moderate loss of central vision
(Page 74, Box 7-2)

Table of Contents

ABOUT CLEVELAND CLINIC'S COLE EYE INSTITUTE

One of the few dedicated and comprehensive eye institutes in the world, Cleveland Clinic's Cole Eye Institute combines research and advanced patient care in a state-of-the-art facility. The Institute's doctors and scientists, all with advanced expertise, draw patients from around the world. Many come because the Institute's highly specialized staff is able to treat the rarest and most complicated cases.

U.S. News & World Report in its annual hospital survey ranks the Cole Eye Institute among the top 10 eye hospitals in the country. The Institute has one of the highest patient volumes in the United States, with more than 192,000 patient visits and 8,000 eye surgeries each year.

Because the Institute combines research with patient care and education, the facility offers patients access to up-to-the-minute technologies, and enables them to participate in clinical trials of the latest treatments. Physicians around the world adopt many eye procedures developed at the Institute. Researchers are now studying the causes of, and developing new treatments for, age-related macular degeneration, glaucoma, diabetic retinopathy, and cataracts. Institute physicians also study and care for the full range of other eye disorders, including pediatric eye problems, cancers of the eye, and refractive errors, such as nearsightedness and farsightedness.

INTRODUCTION

Those who count themselves among the Baby Boom generation are now entering a new phase of life. Retirement looms, and for many in this generation, that means looking forward to some well-deserved rest and relaxation.

While work is becoming a memory for many Baby Boomers, so is clear vision. Most in this generation have to reach for their reading glasses to decipher the Sunday paper. More important, many contend with a variety of eye diseases, from glaucoma to cataracts. At best, these conditions are inconvenient. At worst, these diseases, left undiagnosed and untreated, can steal vision forever.

Most people cannot see as well by age 50 as they did at 20. For some, most of that lost vision will be minor—less contrast and clarity in the dark, and slower adaptation, for example. For others, the changes may be life-changing and disabling. How you anticipate and deal with vision loss will determine whether you can maintain an active lifestyle, or whether you will have to give up many of the activities that you love.

Latest developments in eye research

The goals of this report are to share some of the latest developments in eye research, and to teach you how to preserve your vision so that it won't dramatically affect your life. You will learn how rapidly vision research is progressing. Many illnesses that once blinded people can now be managed with medication, surgery, and a whole range of new therapies. Every day, it seems, scientists announce another new development or breakthrough in eye research—from stem cell therapies to artificial corneas.

Warning signs of vision loss

This report is also designed to alert you to the warning signs of vision loss. Read through them carefully, refer back to this report if you think you might be experiencing symptoms of glaucoma, cataracts, or any other vision problem, and call your ophthalmologist if you are. Taking quick action to find the most appropriate treatment will give you the best chance of preserving your sight today—and into the future.

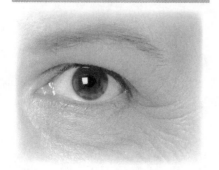

The entire eyeball is only an inch wide—about the size of a walnut.

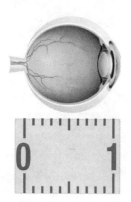

1 ANATOMY OF THE EYE

The human eye is an amazingly complex bit of bioengineering that can focus light and create moving pictures far more efficiently than any camera known to man. It also works with the brain to process and interpret those images more effectively than any digital imaging system yet invented. It's a space saver too: The entire eye is a ball only an inch wide, about the size of a walnut (see Box 1-1, "Size of the eyeball").

Basic structure

Most of the eye is hidden from view, housed in the bony orbit designed to protect it from injury and surrounded by a cushion of fat and muscles that help coordinate its movements (see Box 1-2, "Anatomy of the eye"). When you look at the eye in a mirror, you see the white of the eye, or sclera—a protective coating of collagen that wraps around it. It has an opening in front for the cornea, a clear protective layer that allows light to pass into the eye. The sclera is also interrupted in the back to allow the optic nerve to connect the eye to the brain. There are a few other structures you should know about because they are important to understanding the age-related diseases that can threaten your sight.

Basics of vision

Between the iris and the cornea lies the anterior chamber, which is filled with a clear, watery solution called the aqueous humor. It provides nourishment to the lens and other structures of the anterior chamber, and it removes waste products. The aqueous humor is produced just behind the iris in the ciliary body, whose muscles help the lens change shape. The aqueous flows back toward the lens and eventually out through the pupil to the anterior chamber. In a normal eye, it is drained away through meshwork in the area where the cornea and iris meet. But sometimes the drainage system fails and the aqueous humor builds up. This can lead to an increase in eye pressure, which then damages the optic nerve and causes glaucoma.

The eye is like a camera

You can see the iris, which gives your eye whatever color it has—blue, green, brown, or hazel—and the dark pupil at its center. The iris is like an automatic camera shutter that adjusts the amount of light let into the eye in response to light in the environment. The iris is made of muscle fibers that are constantly in motion, making tiny corrections to expand or contract the pupil, depending on how bright the environment is. The pupil controls how much light enters the eye. It enlarges in dark conditions, and contracts in light conditions.

Behind the iris and pupil is the lens, which helps focus light to form an image on the back wall of the eye. With the help of tiny muscles attached to it, the lens constantly adjusts its shape, functioning much like an automatic camera lens to focus on objects at varying distances.

Light-reactive retina

Behind the lens is a round chamber filled with a gel called the vitreous humor, which gives the eye its shape and allows light to pass through the eye to the retina. Lining the back wall of the eye is the retina, which works like camera film and reacts to light to form an image. The retina is a multi-layered sheet of light-sensitive cells full of different chemicals that react to different wavelengths of light so that we can see different colors and contrast.

ANATOMY OF THE EYE   BOX 1-2

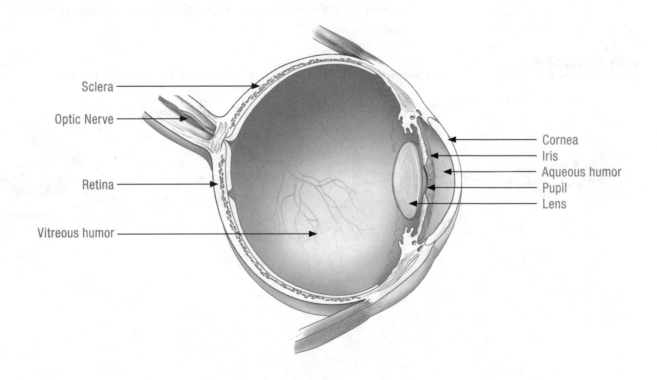

Rods and cones

These photoreceptor cells are called rods and cones. The cones pick up color and are most active in bright light—which is why colors fade and disappear when it gets dark. The cones are also responsible for the finest detail in our central vision, which is why it's hard to read in dim light. Each cone contains a red, yellow, or blue pigment that responds to a range of light wavelengths in that part of the spectrum, enabling us to see an amazing variety of hues and tones.

Most of the cones are located in the macula, a tiny portion of the retina that provides our clearest central vision. The rest of the retina contains mainly rods, which do not perceive color and are responsible for our fuzzier peripheral vision. They also give us night vision and contrast sensitivity.

The rods and cones are connected to other nerve cells that exit the eye through the optic nerve and connect in the brain. Once light signals reach the brain, they are interpreted into the images we perceive.

The choroid

Sandwiched between the retina and the sclera in the back of the eye is a middle layer called the choroid that is packed with blood vessels. These blood vessels help nourish the retina and remove waste. Sometimes, in age-related macular degeneration, choroidal blood vessels grow abnormally, disrupting the retina and causing vision problems.

HOW VISION WORKS

BOX 1-3

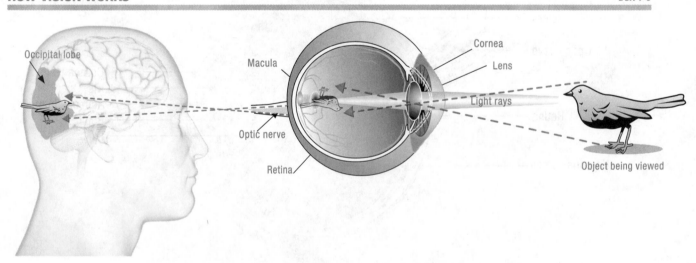

The mechanics of sight

So how do you actually see? When you turn your eyes to look at something, such as a bird, the light waves pass through the cornea, and then through the pupil to the lens, which focuses the image onto your retina by changing its shape. The image is actually projected upside down, and stimulates the rods and cones. They translate the different wavelengths of light into electrical impulses that travel through nerve endings in the retina to the optic nerve, a bundle of about a million nerve cells. The optic nerve carries all that data to the brain, which not only turns the image right side up, but also processes it into a picture you can recognize as a bird. As the bird flies away, subtle changes in the light that bounces off it are reflected on the retina, where they are sent to the brain and interpreted as movement (see Box 1-3, "How vision works").

Anatomical (refractive) errors

Refractive errors are caused when the anatomy, or shape of the eye is distorted in a way that prevents the eye from properly focusing light on the retina. If you wear glasses or contact lenses, you're already familiar with the most common refractive errors, known as nearsightedness, farsightedness and astigmatism (see Box 1-4, "Refractive errors").

REFRACTIVE ERRORS

BOX 1-4

MYOPIA (NEARSIGHTED)	HYPEROPIA (FARSIGHTED)	ASTIGMATISM

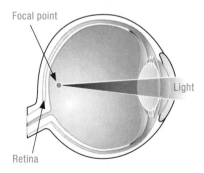

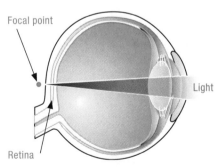

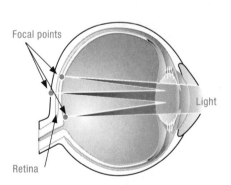

In the nearsighted eye (myopia), light is focused in front of the retina instead of on the retina, causing poor distance vision. In myopes, the eyeball is too long.

In the farsighted eye (hyperopia), light is focused behind the retina, causing poor close-up vision. In hyperopes, the eyeball is too short.

In astigmatism, the shape of the cornea prevents light from focusing properly on the retina, resulting in distortions and blurring of vision. In astigmats, the eyeball is not as symmetric as it should be.

Myopia

Myopia, or nearsightedness, may occur when the eye is longer from front to back than normal, causing the image of distant objects to fall short of the retina instead of focusing precisely on it. A nearsighted person has trouble focusing on distant objects such as street signs, but can see close-up objects clearly.

Hyperopia

Hyperopia, or farsightedness. Hyperopic eyes are often shorter than average, so that images of close objects actually focus behind the retina. A farsighted person can see distant objects clearly but close objects appear fuzzy. As the focusing ability of the lens decreases with age, the problem is further aggravated.

Astigmatism

Astigmatism occurs when the cornea has an oblong shape instead of being round. This decreases its ability to focus light coming from both near and far objects, leading to distorted vision.

Glasses or contact lenses correct these conditions and compensate for distortions by simply bending light before it enters the eye, so the image focuses correctly and sharply on the retina. Refractive corneal surgery can correct refractive errors as well.

2

AGE-RELATED MACULAR DEGENERATION

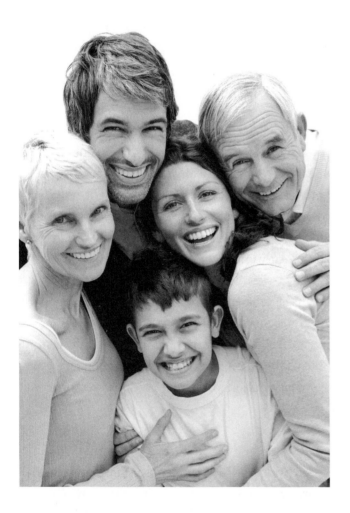
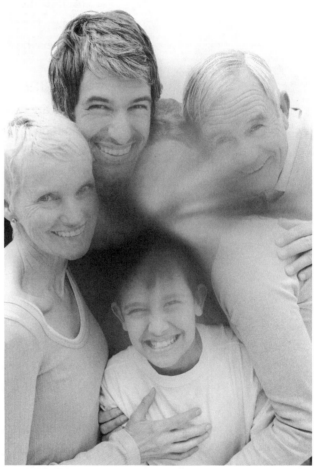

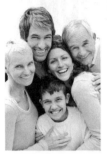 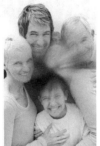

Normal vision   Dry AMD vision

Leading cause of severe vision loss

Age-related macular degeneration (AMD) accounts for more than half of all cases of blindness, and is the leading cause of severe vision loss in Americans over age 65. That's the bad news. Now for the good news—the incidence of the advanced aspects of this sight-robbing disease is on the decline. The prevalence of AMD among adults age 40 and older fell from more than nine percent between in the late 1980s and early 1990s, to 6.5 percent from 2005 to 2008. An estimated 7.2 million Americans have the condition today. Researchers say the reason for the decline in AMD cases is that people are eating better, getting more exercise and not smoking—all of which are contributing to the lower AMD rates. Despite the drop in AMD incidence, however, this disease isn't going away any time soon, which means that older adults still need to be vigilant about their eye health.

Wet and dry AMD

There are two forms of age-related macular degeneration: the more common dry, or non-exudative, form, and the less frequent but far more serious wet, or exudative, form. The dry form is characterized by the slow buildup of products from the breakdown of the light-sensitive cells in the macula, the part of the retina responsible for your sharpest central vision. This form may cause slightly blurred vision (though it often has no symptoms early on), followed by the slow erosion of central vision (see Box 2-1, "Normal vision vs. dry AMD vision").

Over time it may cause a problem with reading or recognizing faces. With dry macular degeneration, drusen—tiny white or yellow deposits—form under the retina. The drusen themselves don't seem to cause blindness, but as they increase, your risk of developing advanced dry macular degeneration or the more serious, wet form of the disease climbs.

A progressive disease

All wet AMD is preceded by dry AMD, and it can develop at any stage of dry AMD, even before symptoms are evident. Unfortunately, researchers do not know the reasons for this progression, and there is no reliable way to tell which dry AMD patients will go on to develop wet AMD. (see Box 2-2, "Normal macula vs. wet and dry macular degeneration"). But based on which characteristics of dry macular disease are present, and their severity, ophthalmologists can predict the likelihood of progression to advanced disease.

Only about 10 percent of all age-related macular degeneration sufferers develop wet AMD, but this form accounts for the majority of blindness from macular degeneration. However, there are now treatments available for wet AMD that may help preserve vision.

Three stages of dry AMD

Stage 1: Almost symptomless

In the early stage, patients have only a few small- or medium-sized drusen and no noticeable symptoms or vision loss.

Stage 2: Vision problems begin

In the intermediate stage, there are many medium-sized drusen or at least one large druse, and patients may begin to notice vision problems. They may have a blurred spot in the center of their vision, or they may need to turn on additional lights in order to read. People

NORMAL MACULA VS. WET AND DRY MACULAR DEGENERATION   BOX 2-2

Enlarged view of the macula under different conditions ...

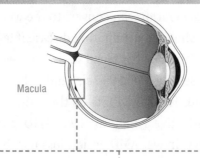

Macula

Normal Macula	Dry AMD	Wet AMD

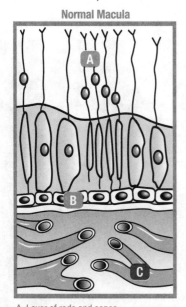 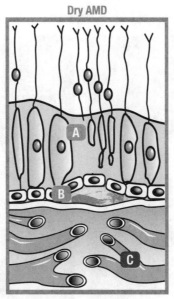 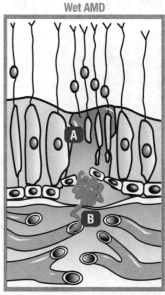

A. Layer of rods and cones (photoreceptors)

B. Retinal pigmented epithelium layer

C. Blood vessels of choroid

A. Degenerating photoreceptors (cell death)

B. Retinal pigmented epithelium layer

C. Drusen

A. Blood

B. New blood vessels

with advanced dry AMD not only have more drusen, but the cells in the macula responsible for detailed vision begin to break down, along with some of the surrounding tissue. This leads to thinning or atrophy of the retina.

Stage 3: Symptoms may become severe

At this stage, symptoms may become severe, and the blurring in the center of the field of vision will grow larger and darker until it becomes difficult to read or see faces.

There is no cure for dry macular degeneration, but certain vitamins and antioxidants may slow its progression. In general, macular degeneration takes many years to compromise vision, and it sometimes doesn't progress at all.

Wet AMD

However, in certain cases, and without warning, dry macular degeneration can convert to the wet form, which is a much faster-moving and debilitating disease if left untreated. In wet or exudative AMD, abnormal blood vessels grow up under the retina. Because these new blood vessels tend to be delicate, they leak blood and other fluid. This liquid lifts up the retina and tends to damage it quickly. A distinctive symptom of wet AMD is that it makes straight lines look wavy. In wet AMD, vision loss may be fast and severe.

NORMAL vs. WET AMD VISION   BOX 2-3

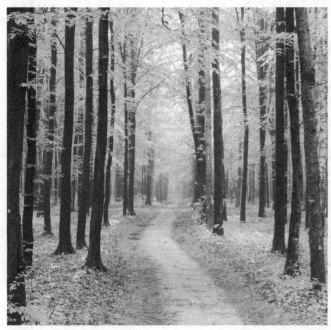

Normal vision

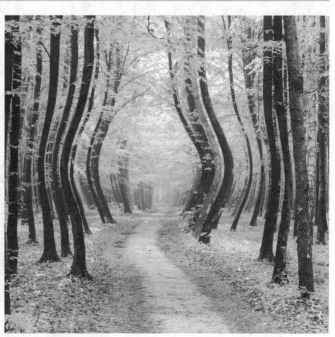

Wet AMD vision

Symptoms of AMD

Because both forms of macular degeneration are painless, vision loss can sneak up on you. Even though the early stages of dry AMD don't cause symptoms, they may lead to the advanced stage or to rapid vision loss from the wet form. The wet form is more likely to be treatable when caught early, and the dry form may be prevented or slowed with certain supplements. That's why it's important to get regular eye exams to catch the disease early—especially if you have a family history of AMD, you smoke, and/or you're overweight. Once vision is lost to macular degeneration, doctors usually cannot restore it.

Subtle first signs

These symptoms (which can be subtle at first) may be signs that you have macular degeneration:

- Increasing need for bright light when reading or doing detailed work
- Blurry vision
- Mildly distorted vision
- Dulling of colors

When symptoms are sudden

With wet macular degeneration, symptoms may appear suddenly and worsen quickly. For that reason, it's important to get to an ophthalmologist right away if you have any of these symptoms:

- Distortions in your central field of vision
- Straight lines that appear wavy or objects that look distorted, caused by the fluid under the retina, are an important early sign of wet AMD (see Box 2-3, "Normal vs. wet AMD vision").
- Blurred vision
- Dulling of colors
- A central blurry spot or blind spot that may be growing (see Box 2-4, "Severe wet AMD vision")
- Difficulty reading
- Trouble recognizing people
- Poor night vision

Advanced macular degeneration usually starts in a single eye but it can affect both eyes at the same time. You may not notice these changes if your other eye compensates, so it's important to check your eyes individually to

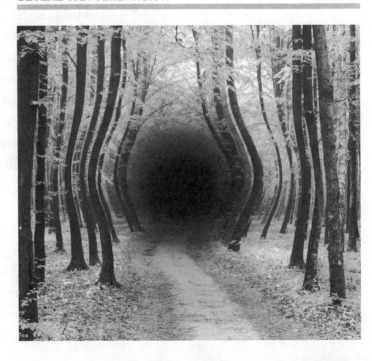

SEVERE WET AMD VISION BOX 2-4

be sure there are no problems. Once you have macular degeneration in one eye, you face a higher risk of it developing in the other eye. You will need to return to your doctor for regular check-ups to monitor how quickly your macular degeneration is progressing.

Causes of macular degeneration

The underlying process of both forms of macular degeneration is thought to be a breakdown in the structures of the retina, but what causes that deterioration isn't well understood. Some researchers think the damaging effects of free radicals and/or low-grade inflammation may be partly to blame. Alternatively, AMD may be caused by the slow starvation of retinal cells, due to the deterioration of cells and structures that deliver nutrition to the retina. Other possible causes:

Genetics

Research has focused on the potential roles of both genetics and inflammation in that process. Investigators have discovered several genes that may be linked to AMD. Variations to two genes—CFH and LOC387715—could help determine whether a person will progress to advanced AMD. A variation of the CFH gene called CFH Y402H might be responsible for more than half of advanced AMD cases in elderly people. AMD also has been linked to variants in the gene for the cytokine, interleukin 8 (IL-8), which is involved with inflammatory processes in the body. Understanding this connection might lead doctors to test patients for the gene in the future, and treat them with anti-inflammatory therapies.

Scientists also have discovered higher levels of C-reactive protein—another marker of inflammation—in people with the CFH genetic variation. Chronic inflammation may be involved in the development of drusen, and it's possible that lowering CRP level might one day reduce the risk of developing this disease.

However, in people who have both genetic variations and who smoke or are overweight, the AMD risk increases 19-fold. Identifying these genetic variations may make it worthwhile to offer genetic testing for people at risk for AMD, so they can modify the risk factors they can control.

Inflammation

Researchers are finding that the health of the eyes is closely tied to the health of other areas of the body, including the mind, kidneys, and vascular system. The same risk factors that predispose people to heart disease, kidney disease and dementia may also make them more likely to develop AMD. People with AMD face more than double the risk of having a heart attack or stroke within 10 years. This may be because the two conditions share not only inflammation, but also other risk factors such as hardening of the arteries (atherosclerosis).

Patients with AMD have a 50 percent higher risk of heart disease than people without AMD. The risk is particularly high in people with specific signs of early AMD, such as soft drusen. Late AMD is not associated with an increased risk for heart disease.

Cystatin C

Patients with high blood levels of cystatin C, a marker of kidney function face an increased risk of AMD, even if they do not have kidney disease. People with AMD might also have a nearly 40 percent greater risk for developing dementia. AMD and dementia (including Alzheimer's disease) may share a similar origin. Both conditions have related vascular risk factors, including high blood pressure and smoking.

Protein interaction

A protein called Roundabout (Robo-4) on the surface of blood vessel cells is thought to affect the formation of the abnormal blood vessels that characterize AMD. Researchers believe that Robo-4 interacts with another protein called Slit2 to prevent the abnormal blood vessel development that occurs in AMD, and in diabetic retinopathy. Drugs that activate the Robo-4 and Slit2 proteins might one day provide another treatment for these conditions.

CFH gene

It's important to note that, although scientists are finding relationships between genes and AMD, genetics don't equate to destiny. Lifestyle also plays an important role in AMD susceptibility. For example, people who have the CFH gene are three times more likely to develop AMD. Those with the LOC387715 genetic variation are four times more likely to get the disease.

Prevention

There is no proven way to prevent age-related macular degeneration, but because some of the risk factors are related to lifestyle, there are changes you can make to reduce your risk of the disease, such as maintaining a healthy weigh and blood pressure control. Lifestyle factors are so important, in fact, that women who introduce a few simple changes could cut their risk of developing AMD by more than two-thirds, according to two large studies from 2010.

Lifestyle factors

Making the appropriate lifestyle changes, whether you have the genetic risk or not, can help you substantially reduce your chances of developing vision loss due to AMD. Age-related macular degeneration typically appears after the age of 50. As you age, the odds go up.

Risk factors you can modify:

- Smoking
- High blood pressure
- High cholesterol
- Dietary factors/ poor nutrition
- Obesity
- Heart disease
- Over-exposure to ultraviolet light

Risk factors you can't modify:

- Caucasian race
- Family history
- Female gender
- Light-colored iris

Supplements: AREDS

The first phase of Age-Related Eye Disease Study (AREDS1), which ended in 2001, led by the National Institutes of Health's National Eye Institute, established that taking high-dose supplements containing vitamin C, vitamin E, beta-carotene, copper and zinc helped slow disease progression in people who were at risk for developing advanced AMD. However, further studies suggested that vitamins C and E are ineffective against AMD.

AREDS 2, which ended in 2011, also found that adding the nutrients lutein and zeaxanthin to the supplements might help retard AMD's progression (see Box 2-5, "Latest results show lutein, zeaxanthin help slow AMD; omega-3s do not"). That result supported the results of an April, 2012 review of nearly 200 scientific papers that the two nutrients may "delay the progress of advanced retinal disease."

Possible side effects of AREDS

There is a small risk of side effects with AREDS type supplements, including anemia, urinary-tract problems and yellowing of the skin. If you are a smoker, you should recall that beta-carotene and vitamin E may slightly increase your risk of developing lung cancer, a finding that was seen once again in AREDS 2. Smokers should not take beta-carotene or vitamin E, either alone or in any AREDS vitamin formulation, because these have been shown to boost the risk of lung cancer. When you talk to your doctor, ask whether this type of supplement is appropriate for you, because it may interact with other vitamin pills you are taking, and it may not be safe if you have or are at risk for certain conditions, such as prostate cancer.

When buying AREDS formulations, check the label carefully because many supplements are advertised as promoting "eye health," yet they may not contain the right vitamins or the correct doses. Only the AREDS formula has been tested in large National Eye Institute-sponsored clinical trials.

Vitamin D and other supplements

Vitamin D might also reduce AMD risk, possibly by reducing inflammation and/or preventing the growth of new blood vessels in the retina, both of which can contribute to the disease. Postmenopausal women with high levels of vitamin D in their blood are much less likely to develop AMD than women with low vitamin D levels, according to a study in the April 11, 2011 *Archives of Ophthalmology*.

That study included more than 1,300 women, ages 50 to 79. In women under age 75, getting at least 720 International Units (IU) of vitamin D from foods and supplements—which is a higher amount than the Institute of Medicine's daily recommendation of 600 IU—correlated to a 59 percent lower AMD risk. The blood concentration of vitamin D in those women was a median of 34 nanograms per milliliter (ng/ml), and ranged from 30 ng/ml to 66 mg/ml. The normal range is 30ng/ml to 74 ng/ml, according to the National Institutes of Health. Because most Americans have insufficient levels of vitamin D, it is a good idea to get your blood tested for vitamin D concentration.

Vitamin B

Evidence also suggests that supplements containing vitamins B6, B12, and folic acid might help prevent AMD. Women who take these supplements daily may reduce their risk of developing the condition by more than 30 percent.

NEW FINDING   BOX 2-5

Latest results show lutein, zeaxanthin help slow AMD; omega-3s do not

The only prophylactic treatment known to reduce the risk of progression and vision loss from age-related macular degeneration is the "AREDS formula," a combination of vitamin and mineral supplements which was studied in the Age-Related Eye Diseases Study (AREDS).

That long-running study originally showed a slowing in disease progression in people at risk for developing advanced AMD among those taking high dose supplements containing vitamins C and E, beta-carotene, copper, and zinc.

Now the latest results, from AREDS-2, suggest that the AREDS supplements formula should be revised to replace the beta-carotene with lutein and zeaxanthin, along with the other ingredients.

The new results also found that adding the omega-3 compounds docosahexaenoic acid (DHA) and eicosapentaenoic acid (EPA) did not slow the progression of AMD. The original AREDS formula was patented and sold by Bausch and Lomb as Ocuvite® PreserVision™.

A second company, Alcon, has licensed sales rights from Bausch and Lomb as well. Updated versions of "AREDS vitamins" were scheduled to come to market in the second half of 2013. Most likely, the updated formula will include 400 IU of vitamin E, 500 mg of vitamin C, 10 mg lutein, 2 mg zeaxanthin, 80 mg zinc, and 2 mg copper. When buying such supplements, check these quantities on the label.

Journal of the American Medical Association, May 5, 2013

Diagnosis for wet or dry AMD

Macular degeneration is usually diagnosed using a standard dilated eye exam, in which the ophthalmologist will check your retina for signs of damage. The doctor will look for drusen, as well as a mottled appearance of the macula, which normally appears uniform.

Tests for wet AMD

Amsler grid

He or she will also give you a simple test called the Amsler grid to check for signs that you have developed wet AMD. This test uses a chart that looks similar to a piece of graph paper. If you notice wavy, broken or distorted lines on the graph, the doctor will note their location and the degree of distortion to determine where the damage to your macula is located, as well as its extent.

If you are diagnosed with either form of AMD, ask your doctor for a copy of the Amsler grid and use it to check your eyes individually every day. If you have dry AMD, this can help you catch the conversion to wet AMD at an early stage, when it is more likely to be treatable. If you have wet AMD, be aware that many treatments need to be repeated as they wear off, or as new areas of abnormal blood vessels develop. The grid can help you identify when your symptoms have returned and you need another treatment.

To use the Amsler grid at home (see Box 2-6, "Amsler grid"), cover one eye and look at the grid, then switch and cover the other eye. If you detect any changes in the grid's appearance, call your ophthalmologist immediately to get a dilated eye exam.

You may need additional testing to determine whether you have wet AMD. Other tests include a fluorescein angiogram and an optical coherence tomography (OCT) scan.

Fluroscein angiogram

A fluorescein angiogram involves injecting fluorescent dye into your arm. The dye passes through the blood vessels in your retina, making the normal and abnormal blood vessels easier for the doctor to see. The doctor will take a picture of your retina as the dye passes through so he can detect any leaking blood vessels and determine the best treatment.

Optical coherence tomography

In OCT scanning, you will be asked to sit at a machine that looks something like a slit lamp and look straight ahead at a target. The machine will take cross-sectional images of your retina based on the reflection of light and/or ultrasound waves.

AMSLER GRID BOX 2-6

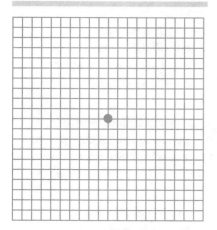

Amsler grid as seen by a person without AMD.

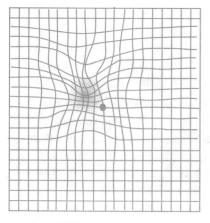

Amsler grid as seen by a person with AMD.

Researchers are also investigating a computer-based method that evaluates the eye's ability to distinguish details and shapes of objects. The test can compare a person's visual acuity before surgery or visual rehabilitation to the acuity after treatment to see how well treatments are working. It might also help doctors diagnose AMD sooner.

Treatment for dry AMD

There is no treatment for dry AMD that can reverse vision loss once it reaches the advanced atrophic stage. Fortunately, early and intermediate dry AMD are usually slow to progress, and many people live normal lives with few vision problems for many years. You will need to monitor the condition using the Amsler grid, and have regular eye exams to be sure the disease isn't progressing or developing into wet AMD.

Treatment for wet AMD
Anti-angiogenesis compounds

There has been a dramatic improvement in treatments for wet AMD over the past few years with the use of anti-angiogenesis compounds. These drugs, which were originally designed to treat cancer, work by blocking the formation of new blood vessels and slowing the leakage of blood into the eye, and they are the first treatments that can actually improve vision for some patients. The older anti-angiogenesis drugs are Lucentis (ranibizumab) and Avastin (bevacizumab), and their use is on the rise. Since 2001, the number of people receiving Lucentis and Avastin injections has doubled each year. The U.S. Food and Drug Administration approved a new effective and safe anti-angiogenesis drug, Eylea (VEGF Trap-Eye), for wet AMD in November 2011. Since then, the number of prescriptions for Eylea has also risen rapidly.

Lucentis

Ranibizumab (Lucentis) is injected into the eye once a month. It targets vascular endothelial growth factor (VEGF), a protein that triggers angiogenesis. Clinical trials have found that Lucentis stabilizes vision in more than 90 percent of patients and even improves it in roughly 30 percent of patients. The main side effects with Lucentis are inflammation and infection, but these are rare. There is also a small risk of retinal detachment, bleeding, eye pain, increased eye pressure, cataract and floaters. The good news is that Lucentis doesn't appear to increase the risk for heart problems. In fact, patients treated with this drug may face a lower risk of

Lucentis works better on wet AMD when combined with Fovista

Two different inhibitors of new vascular growth are considerably more effective when used together than is Lucentis alone against wet age-related macular degeneration, according to a study that was presented at the November, 2012 annual meeting of the American Academy of Ophthalmology. Patients receiving combination therapy gained a mean of 10.6 letters of vision, compared to 6.5 letters for those on Lucentis alone.

Along with Lucentis, patients on dual therapy received the experimental drug, Fovista, which targets both platelet-derived growth factor (PDGF) and vascular endothelial growth factor (VEGF). An anti-PDGF agent renders the neovascular complex more vulnerable to Lucentis, so the drug combination "makes good physiologic sense," Pravin U. Dugel, MD, a clinical associate professor at the Doheny Eye Institute at the Keck School of Medicine, University of Southern California, Los Angeles, said in a press briefing at the meeting. No new adverse events related to the new drug were reported during the clinical trial.

Nonetheless, the study was a Phase 2b study, which is only the second of three stages of clinical trials that precede drug approval decisions by the FDA.

heart attack and heart-related death than patients treated with photodynamic therapy, Macugen, or the other VEGF blocker, Avastin.

One big drawback to Lucentis is its price—a single dose costs around $2,000. The use of Lucentis for treating AMD is covered by most insurance policies. However, Avastin offers a lower-cost alternative.

Fovista

The experimental drug, Fovista targets both platelet-derived growth factor (PDGF) and vascular endothelial growth factor (VEGF) (see Box 2-7, "Lucentis works better on wet AMD when combined with Fovista").

Avastin

Avastin, another VEGF blocker, has shown promise for improving visual acuity in people with wet AMD, and it is much less expensive than Lucentis—about $50 per dose. That's likely why more than half of Medicare patients with AMD who are prescribed a biologic drug today take Avastin instead of Lucentis, according to research reported at the 2010 American Academy of Ophthalmology meeting.

Though Avastin is not FDA-approved for AMD, doctors may legally prescribe a drug for a different use once the FDA has approved it. The two drugs are very similar—Lucentis is a derivative of Avastin formulated specifically for use in the eye. In fact, two studies published in April and May 2012, respectively, found these two drugs to be highly, and equally, effective, with patients gaining a mean of 8.8 letters and 7.8 letters on Lucentis and Avastin, respectively. In addition to showing comparability of the two drugs, the studies also showed that less-frequent treatments were as effective as monthly injections, although monthly monitoring is needed. An important difference between the two drugs is cost: about $50 per dose for Avastin vs. Lucentis' $2,000.

Eylea

In clinical trials, Eylea (VEGF Trap-Eye) was as effective as Lucentis, and after three initial doses, has a more convenient bimonthly dosing schedule. It was also considered equally safe, and approved specifically for wet AMD. Like Lucentis and Avastin, it blocks VEGF, but the mechanism is slightly different from that of the other two drugs (see Box 2-8, "Three treatment options for wet AMD").

BOX 2-8

Macugen

In addition to Lucentis, Avastin, and VEGF Trap-Eye, there are older treatment options available for wet AMD. These older options have limitations—they are less effective and only slow vision loss, rather than halting it, or improving vision that's already deteriorated.

One of the options is pegaptanib sodium (Macugen), which is injected directly into the eye every six weeks to help stabilize and slow vision loss. Macugen was the first anti-angiogenesis drug for the eye. It doesn't work for everyone, and it doesn't improve vision as well as Lucentis or Avastin, but the drug does seem to slow or stabilize vision loss in most patients who take it.

Side effects of Macugen include infection, injury to the lens of the eye and retinal detachment. To prevent infection, your doctor may prescribe antibiotic drops after the injection.

Photodynamic therapy

Another option for wet AMD is photodynamic therapy, which works for some patients who are not eligible for anti-VEGF therapy, or may be used along with anti-VEGF therapy. Photodynamic therapy uses a combination of a non-thermal laser and a light-sensitizing drug to target the abnormal blood vessels while sparing healthy tissue. Long-term studies on photodynamic therapy have shown that the treatment is safe. However, a study in the January 2010 issue of the *Archives of Ophthalmology* finds that it doesn't add to the effectiveness of medication treatment for AMD, or reduce the need for injections with Lucentis. As doctors increasingly turn to Lucentis, Eylea, and Avastin, the number of people using photodynamic therapy is dropping, down 83 percent between 1997 and 2007 and to even lower rates now.

Painless procedure

Photodynamic therapy is a relatively painless procedure that takes about 40 minutes in a doctor's office. First, the drug Visudyne (verteporfin) is injected into your arm. It travels through your body and, when it reaches your eye, it accumulates in the abnormal blood vessels. Your doctor will activate the drug by shining a non-thermal laser into your eye for about 90 seconds. The activated drug will destroy the abnormal blood vessels, leaving the rods, cones and the retina above it relatively untouched. Because the drug is activated by light, you must

Three treatment options for wet AMD

The new drug, Eylea (also called VEGF Trap-Eye) appears to be as effective, broadly speaking, as Lucentis, according to a literature review in the August 2012 *American Journal of Ophthalmology,* and to two major clinical studies published together in the December 2012 issue of *Ophthalmology*. Before Eylea came to market, two drugs were available for wet AMD, Lucentis and Avastin, which most doctors view as offering similar outcomes.

Outcomes on Eylea matched those on monthly doses of Lucentis, even with only bimonthly dosing after the first three (monthly) doses. Bimonthly dosing of Lucentis has not been tested, and currently, Lucentis requires monthly monitoring even when it is given on an as-needed basis. Eylea is slightly less expensive than Lucentis.

BOTTOM LINE

While statistically Eylea and Lucentis have very similar efficacy, either one may be significantly better for you. Now there are two good FDA-approved options for age-related macular degeneration—a good thing. Avastin, widely used for age-related macular degeneration, and approved for other, non-eye-related indications, but not for AMD, is a third, and is less costly.

avoid sunlight or even bright indoor halogen lights for about two days after the procedure until the drug clears your body (the FDA label advises sunlight avoidance for three to five days, but in practice, most all eye doctors are comfortable suggesting two or even one day of sunlight avoidance). You also may be more sensitive to light than usual.

As with laser treatments and anti-angiogenesis drugs, photodynamic therapy requires repeat treatments. You will have to be vigilant about monitoring your condition at home and going to the doctor for frequent follow-ups. An Australian study of photodynamic therapy found that patients who failed to get frequent follow-ups were no better off after a year than if they hadn't gone through the treatment.

Laser photocoagulation

Another treatment for wet AMD is laser photocoagulation, which was once the only option available for the condition. Only about 15 percent of patients are good candidates for this procedure, which uses a laser to seal leaking blood vessels. Your doctor will use a fluorescein angiogram to assess the location and characteristics of the new blood vessels to determine whether this is a viable option for you. Laser surgery works best on newly formed blood vessels that are not growing into the center of the fovea (the center of the macula).

Brief surgery

Laser surgery takes about 30 minutes in an ophthalmologist's office. The doctor will focus a laser directly onto the abnormal blood vessels to destroy them. Unfortunately, the laser surgeon will likely have to burn through part of the retina to get to them, which will also destroy healthy retinal tissue. You may have slight discomfort and sensitivity to light after surgery.

This treatment works permanently in only about half of patients. The remainder will need to repeat the laser surgery, or need some of the previously mentioned treatments because the vessels will begin to grow again, particularly if they recur in the central macula. If you carefully monitor your condition and return to your doctor for frequent check-ups, you will probably retain more of your vision than if you skip treatment.

New treatments

In the past, 90 percent of patients lost vision if they had wet AMD; now about 90 percent can remain stable with treatment and about one-third may improve. Though macular degeneration is a difficult disease, there is even more hope for the future. Many companies are working on new drugs to treat it. Surgeons are perfecting procedures, and medical device companies are working on tiny telescopes or even bionic eyes that might one day restore sight to the blind. One device that is a reality today is an Implantable Miniature Telescope (IMT), which the FDA approved in July 2010 to help patients with late-stage AMD see more clearly. When this device is implanted in one eye, it replaces the eye's natural lens and magnifies images two or more times. Because the IMT can damage corneal cells, it is only recommended for patients age 75 or older with severe vision loss.

Researchers also are investigating a drug that can turn off, or "silence," the genes that lead to wet AMD. This first-of-its kind treatment, called bevasiranib, turns off the gene responsible for the production of vascular endothelial growth factor (VEGF), which is believed to stimulate the growth of abnormal blood vessels in wet AMD. It can halt new blood vessel growth for more than three months after an injection. Bevasiranib not only appears to stabilize patients' vision, but it also improves vision in about a third of patients who receive it.

One treatment that could dramatically change the future outlook for patients with AMD is embryonic stem cell therapy. Though controversial, this treatment could potentially offer a cure for AMD. In an important step forward, the FDA has approved the very first clinical trial of embryonic stem cell therapy for AMD. During the study, 12 patients with the dry form of AMD will receive implants of 50,000 to 200,000 cells underneath their retina. The hope is that these cells will repair the damaged retina and restore lost vision.

3 COMMON CONDITIONS OF THE AGING EYE

Aging eye (presbyopia)

The most common age-related vision problem is presbyopia (far-sightedness), which sooner or later requires nearly everyone to adopt reading glasses or bifocals. Presbyopia occurs when the lens loses some of its flexibility as it ages and can no longer change its shape sufficiently to focus on close objects. It's a gradual, natural, and inevitable process that may begin as early as your 20s and progress until you need corrective lenses, usually sometime in your 40s (see Box 3-1, "Normal vision vs. aging eye (presbyopia)").

If you have presbyopia, you may first notice that you have difficulty reading at your normal distance, or you develop headaches or eyestrain when reading or doing close work. You tend to hold things farther away to read them. When this becomes a problem (your arms are not long enough), your doctor can diagnose the condition with a simple eye exam. Presbyopia can be solved with reading glasses or contact lenses if you already wear glasses.

Presbyopia treatment options
Corrective lenses

▶ Bifocals: These are glasses that correct both distance vision and reading vision. Typically, there is a horizontal line across the middle of the lens. They correct your distance vision when you look through the upper part of the lens. When you look through the

---

NORMAL VISION VS. AGING EYE (PRESBYOPIA)   BOX 3-1

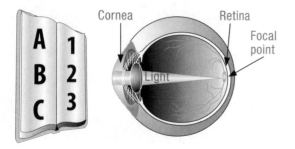

With normal vision, the lens focuses properly at the back of the retina.

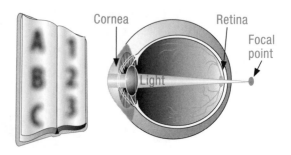

With presbyopia, the lens loses its flexibility and can no longer change shape sufficiently to focus on close objects.

lower part of the lens, they allow you to read clearly. Progressive bifocals are similar, but they don't have a line in the middle and the lens correction varies as you look through different aspects of the lens, which is set for distance vision at the top, intermediate vision (for example, to see objects at arm's length) in the middle, and for reading at the bottom. Bifocal contact lenses are available for people who wear contacts, and multifocal lens implants are available for patients having cataract surgery.

▶ Trifocals: These lenses correct for distance vision, middle-distance vision (such as looking at your computer screen), and close-up vision.

▶ Monovision correction: This type of correction uses a contact lens for distance vision in one eye and a lens for close-up work in the other. Although it takes some getting used to, monovision can restore nearly perfect vision with one eye optimized for distance and the other for near. Some patients love monovision while others hate it.

Laser options

Glasses and contact lenses aren't the only options for treating refractive errors. Laser surgery techniques have transformed vision correction:

▶ An implanted multifocal lens

This lens can function like a younger eye, adjusting between near and far objects to provide clear vision at all distances (see Box 3-2, "Multifocal lens"). During surgery, the natural lens of the eye is removed and then replaced with the artificial lens. Multifocal lenses can reduce and may eliminate the need for contacts or glasses. Some patients may have difficulty with glare and image resolution with these lenses.

MULTIFOCAL LENS   BOX 3-2

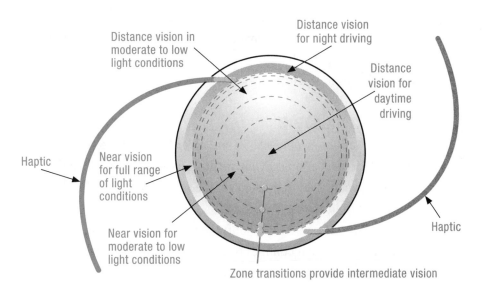

Distance vision in moderate to low light conditions
Distance vision for night driving
Distance vision for daytime driving
Haptic
Near vision for full range of light conditions
Near vision for moderate to low light conditions
Zone transitions provide intermediate vision
Haptic

Multifocal lens implants can help you see better at all distances—close up, and far away.

Multifocal (intraocular) lens: The circular clear disc is the lens optic. The dark orange lines on either side of the optic are called the "haptics." They help hold the lens in the correct position in the eye.

▶ LASIK or PRK

These procedures, laser-assisted in situ keratomileusis (LASIK) or photorefractive keratectomy (PRK), reshape the eye so that it provides better near vision for reading and other close tasks, although this usually means you will require eyeglasses for distance. It has become a very common surgical technique, and most patients say they are satisfied with the results of their LASIK surgery.

Nearsightedness (myopia)

Myopia (see Box 3-3, "Myopia") affects an estimated 32 million people age 40 and older in the United States. Glasses, contact lenses, and LASIK are all effective treatments. Other options include:

▶ "Phakic" intraocular lens (IOL) implant. In this procedure, an artificial lens is implanted into the eye and the natural lens is left in place. Although the intraocular lens implant is safe and effective based on study outcomes, more research is still needed to determine whether there may be any long-term complications from the procedure, such as cataracts or glaucoma. This option is a consideration, particularly for patients who don't qualify for LASIK.

▶ CustomVue Monovision LASIK: This procedure treats one eye for myopia and the other for presbyopia. Monovision procedures are a lot like wearing monovision contacts—you can see at a distance out of one eye and close-up out of the other. Usually you can adapt to this and won't notice it, though it may take as long as six to eight weeks to do so. The American Academy of Ophthalmology recommends that you try monovision contact lenses before you commit to surgery, so you know whether you can adjust to permanent monovision.

Even after surgery, in some cases you may still need glasses in certain situations, such as driving. Also, it's quite possible that your eyes will continue to change as you age, and you may end up needing reading glasses in the future.

Dry eye syndrome

Nearly five million people age 50 and older have dry eye syndrome, according to the National Eye Institute. Dry eye occurs when the eyes don't produce enough tears, or the tears don't have the right consistency to lubricate the eye.

Women who have gone through menopause are at greatest risk because the hormonal changes that occur during menopause reduce tear production and subtly increase inflammation in the eye. Older

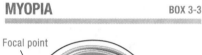

MYOPIA　　　　　　　BOX 3-3

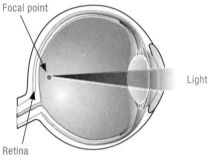

In the nearsighted eye, light is focused in front of the retina instead of on the retina, causing poor distance vision.

BOX 3-4

men are also at risk, especially if they have high blood pressure or benign prostate growth. About 1.68 million men age 50 and over have dry eye syndrome, and the prevalence is expected to rise to 2.79 million by the year 2030. Declining male hormone levels may contribute to the deterioration of the tear film, which provides moisture and protection to the front of the eye. Other risk factors include overuse of the eyes (such as using a computer or driving a lot), smoking, LASIK surgery, and long-term use of contact lenses.

Eye dryness causes irritation that stimulates a rush of tears, so you may actually experience dry eye as an overly watery eye that is prone to irritation and tearing. However, the watery tears may be deficient in certain components and do not sooth the eyes effectively. Symptoms include aching, redness, stinging, burning, itchiness, and the sense that there's something in your eye. Many people ignore these symptoms, not realizing they have a treatable medical condition. Untreated dry eye syndrome is more than a mere annoyance—it can have profound effects on your everyday life, and it can eventually threaten your sight.

Treatment options for dry eye syndrome

Even when it is relatively mild, dry eye syndrome is uncomfortable, but in most cases it can easily be treated with over-the-counter artificial tears. You may need to try drops with different formulations to see which one works for you. Eye drops containing omega-3 fatty acids might help reduce the inflammation in dry eye. For patients who don't respond to conventional dry eye treatments, drops containing the immune-suppressing anti-inflammatory drug cyclosporine may offer some symptom relief.

Severe dry eye

More severe cases may be treated by inserting tiny plugs into your eye's drainage system to block tear flow from your eye into your nose. These plugs force your natural tears to back up into your eye, which can help maintain moisture. Another new option for treating dry eye is a prescription medicated insert (Lacrisert) that dissolves in the eye to provide lubrication. And a study in the May 2012 issue of *Ophthalmology* found that caffeine can boost tear production, raising the possibility that the compound might prove helpful for patients with dry eye syndrome.

See Box 3-4, "Dry eye preventive strategies," for some simple preventive strategies to help keep your eyes moist if you have dry eye syndrome.

Dry eye preventive strategies

Here are some simple preventive strategies to help keep your eyes moist if you have dry eye syndrome:

- Use a humidifier in your home to increase moisture in the air.
- Wear glasses that wrap around your face or have side shields to prevent wind from evaporating your natural tears.
- When using the computer, reading or focusing on other tasks, take breaks, look away and deliberately blink periodically. While concentrating, we often forget to blink as often as we should.

BOX 3-5

Other age-related eye problems
Floaters

These are the tiny specks or cobwebs that seem to float across your eye. They normally increase as you age and are rarely serious. However, if the number of floaters increases dramatically and/or suddenly, particularly if you notice flashes of light as they occur, seek immediate medical attention. This can be a sign of retinal tearing or detachment, which can permanently harm your vision.

Corneal conditions

Disease, infection or injury can damage the cornea—the clear dome at the front of your eye. You may experience symptoms such as redness, watery eyes, pain, reduced vision or a halo effect around objects. Your doctor can treat these problems with a new eyeglass prescription, eye drops or, in severe cases, surgery.

Conjunctivitis

Conjunctivitis, or pink eye. This common eye condition causes itching, burning or tearing and is usually caused by allergies or an infection. You can treat viral conjunctivitis with cool compresses and artificial tears. Antibiotic eye drops can relieve bacterial conjunctivitis. Antibacterial drugs work against many of the bacteria that cause conjunctivitis. Allergic conjunctivitis can be treated with anti-allergic eye drops.

Eyelid problems

Some diseases and conditions, such as rosacea, can cause problems with the eyelids, leading to pain, itching, tearing or sensitivity to light. You can usually treat these conditions with medicine or by carefully cleansing the lids (lid scrub).

Routine care

The eye is incredibly hardy, but with so many complicated, coordinating parts, it's almost inevitable that problems occur. As you age, your odds of developing an eye condition increase dramatically, and you become more prone to the four biggest age-related diseases: macular degeneration, cataracts, glaucoma, and diabetic retinopathy. Because symptoms may not appear until one of these diseases has progressed too far to treat, your best defense is to get regular and thorough eye exams.

If you don't have any signs of, or risk factors for, eye disease, the American Academy of Ophthalmology recommends that you have a baseline eye exam at age 40 (see Box 3-5, "What to expect at your eye exam"). Your ophthalmologist will recommend the interval at which you should have regular eye exams after that, based on your risk factors. By age 65, you should schedule an exam every one to two years with an ophthalmologist.

People who are at greater risk for certain eye conditions should have their eyes examined more often than is recommended for otherwise healthy people. These include people with diabetes (who are at high risk for diabetic retinopathy), African-Americans (who are at greater risk for developing glaucoma) and people with a family history of eye disease or a personal history of developmental delay, premature birth, high blood pressure, HIV or previous eye injury. If you have any concerns about your risks, discuss the need for more frequent eye exams with your ophthalmologist.

Eye exam

Many people get their eyes examined by optometrists at discount outlets. This type of exam is fine to determine your eyeglass prescription or pick up new contact lenses, but it's generally not thorough enough to screen for age-related eye diseases, because many of these eye care providers don't dilate your eyes with drops. Dilating the eyes expands the pupil, and it's a crucial step in checking for the early signs of eye disease, because it gives the doctor a much better view of what's going on inside your eye.

In addition to checking your vision with the standard Snellen eye chart (see Box 3-6, "Snellen eye chart"), an eye exam (see Box 3-7, "Eye exam") should include a test of your peripheral vision, a retinal

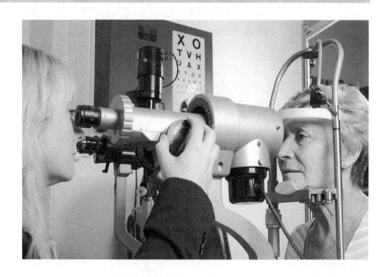

You should have a baseline eye exam at age 40, and every one to two years after age 65.

The exam should include a standard vision check, a test of your peripheral vision, a retinal exam, an eye pressure test as part of a check for glaucoma and an examination of your inner eye.

exam and a test of eye pressure as part of a check for glaucoma. The eye exam should also include a thorough review of your inner eye.

For more information, see Resources on page 80.

Don't ignore these symptoms

Many people overlook the early signs of serious eye disease because the symptoms are painless, or seem too minor to bother checking out. As a result, patients don't get help in the early stages of their disease, when treatments are most effective. Symptoms of serious eye disease can include:

▶ Difficulty adjusting to changes in light, such as trouble seeing in dark rooms or unusual sensitivity to bright light or glare
▶ Spots or shadows in front of your eyes
▶ Dryness, itching or burning
▶ Excessive tearing
▶ Lines that appear distorted or wavy
▶ Double vision
▶ A dark spot in the center of your field of view
▶ Eye pain
▶ Swollen or encrusted lids
▶ A change in eye color
▶ Difficulty focusing
▶ Sudden loss of vision in one eye
▶ Sudden hazy or blurred vision
▶ Flashes of light in front of your eyes
▶ Colored circles that appear around lights
▶ Loss of peripheral vision
▶ Partial loss of vision

So that you don't needlessly lose your vision, see an eye doctor if you experience any of these symptoms, or any other symptoms that seem unusual, new or of concern.

4
CATARACTS

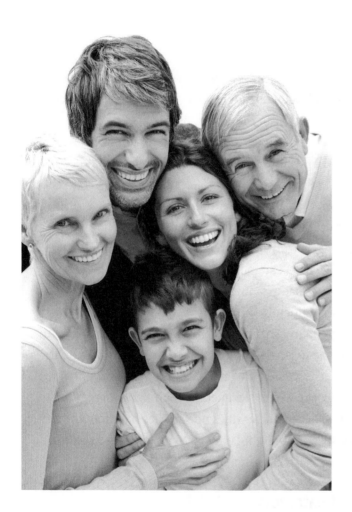

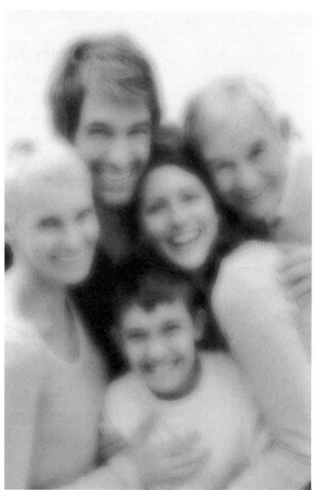

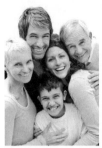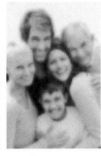

Normal vision   Vision with a
                       Cataract

Cataracts: most common cause of low vision

A Cataracts are the leading cause of blindness in the world. Here in the United States, where we have access to surgery, they rarely lead to complete blindness. However, they are still the most common cause of low vision. Cataracts affect more than 20 million Americans over age 40, according to the Centers for Disease Control and Prevention. The risk of cataracts rapidly increases as people age—more than half of everyone over age 80 has a cataract. With the aging of the population, it's estimated that by the year 2020, 30 million Americans will have cataracts.

Cloudy lens

A cataract is a clouding of the eye's lens. The clear lens is made up mostly of protein and water, arranged in a very precise pattern so that light passes through it to the retina. As you age, the lens undergoes natural changes, and the proteins begin to clump, causing the lens to cloud and turn yellow. This is a normal process that occurs in almost everyone, and it doesn't always affect sight. However, in about half the population, the cataract eventually gets so cloudy that it begins to blur or dull vision. The clouded lens scatters light, preventing it from focusing sharply on the retina (see Box 4-1, "Normal vision vs. to vision with a cataract"). It may also cast a yellow or brown tint over your vision, fading colors and contrast as it worsens, and making reading difficult.

Scientists are not sure what causes the clumping associated with cataracts; it could be normal wear and tear in the eye as we age. It also may be damage caused by free radicals, the "loose cannons" of the molecular world, which ricochet through tissue over time and damage cells. This could be why some studies have found that smoking or exposure to sunlight is linked to an increased risk of cataracts—both are sources of free radicals.

Three types of cataracts

There are three types of cataracts. Nuclear cataracts, which form in the center of the lens, are the most common age-related cataracts. Cortical cataracts occur at the edge of the lens and then progress toward the center. Posterior subcapsular cataracts form at the back of the lens and are more common with injury, long-term steroid use, or diabetes.

Risk factors

Everyone is at risk for cataracts as they age, but some people have greater odds of getting them than others. For example, women are more likely to develop cataracts than men. Women who receive hormone replacement therapy (HRT) after menopause are more likely to need cataract surgery than women who are not on HRT, especially if they also drink more than one alcoholic drink per day. The types of estrogens used in HRT may raise levels of C-reactive protein—an inflammatory substance that has been linked to cataract development. Smoking also increases the cataract risk, and it can take 10 to 20 years after kicking the habit for your risk to drop.

Certain medications

Taking certain medications may also make you more prone to developing cataracts. Examples are steroid drugs, like those contained in many common asthma medications, as well as a class of antidepressants known as selective serotonin reuptake inhibitors (SSRIs).

A recent study found that taking the SSRI fluvoxamine (Luvox) was associated with a 51 percent higher risk of having cataract surgery, and taking venlafaxine (Effexor) correlated to a 34 percent higher risk. There didn't appear to be a higher risk with the SSRI drugs fluoxetine (Prozac), citalopram (Celexa), and sertraline (Zoloft). Other risk factors for cataracts include:

- Diabetes
- A family history of cataracts
- A history of eye injury
- Previous eye surgery
- Smoking
- High exposure to sunlight
- High exposure to radiation

Prevention

There is no scientifically proven method to prevent cataracts because most are the unavoidable consequence of aging, and some people may have an inherent genetic susceptibility to them as well.

However, there are some healthy lifestyle changes you can make that may reduce your risks. When you are outside, it's a good idea to wear sunglasses and/or a hat with a brim to limit your exposure to sunlight. When choosing sunglasses, go with function over fashion. Many sunglasses on the market look good, but do little to protect your eyes from the harmful rays of the sun.

Here's what to look for in a pair of sunglasses:

- Sunglasses should block 99 to 100 percent of UVA and UVB rays, because both are harmful.

- **Sunglasses should be dark** enough to reduce glare (however, a darker lens doesn't necessarily mean the glasses block more ultraviolet light).
- **Wrap-around sunglasses** can prevent light from entering the sides of your eyes (for maximum protection, you should also wear a hat with a wide brim).
- **Don't depend on polarized** or mirrored sunglasses. Although these lenses may help block glare, by themselves they do not protect against UV light.

Other preventative steps

- **Stop smoking**
- **Reduce your alcohol** consumption if you drink heavily
- **If you have diabetes,** follow your doctor's instructions and keep tight control of your blood sugar levels
- **Eat a healthy diet** with at least two-and-a-half cups of fruit and two cups of vegetables a day

Vitamin supplements

You may have seen vitamin supplements that claim to prevent eye diseases, including cataracts. To date, the research on these supplements has been inconclusive, and although some studies suggest they might be helpful, there isn't any solid evidence that they work. The Age-Related Eye Disease Study (AREDS), a large and scientifically rigorous research effort conducted by the National Eye Institute, found no benefit to supplementing with high doses of vitamins E and C and beta-carotene for the prevention of cataracts.

The new AREDS 2 study, highlighted in Chapter 2, which also looked at cataract prevention, again saw no benefit to the supplements (see page 21). The Physicians' Health Study II also found no benefit to vitamin C and E supplements. That study included more than 14,000 male doctors and stretched over an average of eight years.

However, the researchers say that given the slow rate at which cataracts develop, the study's duration might have been too short to enable the vitamins to have an effect. Other research has suggested that there might be some benefit to taking the nutrients lutein, niacin, thiamin, and riboflavin, but this hasn't yet been confirmed.

Statins

There is some evidence that statins, the cholesterol-lowering drugs, might help prevent cataracts. More than one study has found that people who take these drugs have a significantly lower risk of developing cataracts than people who don't take statins. Incidentally, statin use may reduce the chance of glaucoma diagnosis as well.

Symptoms

The most common symptoms of a cataract are:

▸ Cloudy or blurry vision—as if you were looking through a dirty windshield
▸ Colors that seem faded or dull
▸ Increased glare from lamps, sunlight and headlights, or circles or halos forming around lights at night
▸ Reduced night vision
▸ Double vision that does not disappear when the other eye is closed
▸ Frequent prescription changes in your glasses or contacts
▸ Increased nearsightedness
▸ Reduced ability to judge contrast
▸ Need for more light for reading or detailed work

Diagnosis

Cataracts are painless and develop slowly, so symptoms may not be noticeable or alarming at first. If you do have any of the symptoms listed above, you should see an ophthalmologist. Your doctor will do a standard dilated eye exam, complete with a slit lamp examination of the lens, to determine whether you have a cataract and how extensive it is. Your doctor should also do the full battery of tests to rule out other eye diseases that can cause similar symptoms.

Treatment

Once you have been diagnosed with a visually significant cataract, the only proven treatment is surgery. If your vision is not yet seriously impaired or does not interfere with your daily life, you may be able to wait to have surgery and correct your vision with glasses or contact lenses. Cataracts may progress slowly, and many people successfully avoid surgery for years—or never need it. This is particularly true of older people, who tend to have slower-growing cataracts.

Risks

Night driving

Cataracts can make night driving hazardous. Some people with cataracts may have difficulty recognizing pedestrians at night, according to a study published online in *Investigative Ophthalmology*

Cataract "holiday"

Ironically, sometimes cataracts actually cause a temporary vision improvement, called a cataract "holiday," in people who wear glasses or contacts before their vision worsens

Cataract surgery associated with reduced hip fractures

Cataract patients who had surgery were 16 percent less likely than control subjects who had cataracts, but no cataract surgery, to suffer hips fractures within a year of surgery. The study included roughly 400,000 Medicare beneficiaries, who were 65 and older.

People with impaired vision are known to be more likely to suffer fractures, according to the study, which was published August 1, 2012 in the *Journal of the American Medical Association*. Nonetheless, it is not clear how much of the reduced risk of hip fracture might be due to improved vision following surgery, and how much might be due to other factors, such as (hypothetically) better general health and/or greater physical activity among those who opt for surgery.

& Visual Science March 16, 2012. In the study, research participants wearing special lenses designed to simulate vision with cataracts had to be five times closer to pedestrians to recognize them as such than those without the special lenses.

Waiting to have cataract surgery following diagnosis may be risky for other reasons. Certain conditions, such as diabetes, can cause cataracts to grow more rapidly. People who wait several months to have surgery may have more problems with vision loss and falls than those who opt for surgery within a few weeks after being diagnosed.

Cataract surgery is successful at improving vision more than 90 percent of the time, and major complications are rare, occurring in about 1-2% of surgeries. But as with all surgery, there are risks, discomfort, and inconvenience. Among the most common complications are mild high blood pressure and mild irregular heartbeat. Other risks include bleeding and swelling of the retina, eye infection, or retinal detachment (an urgent situation that can lead to blindness if not treated quickly). Have a detailed discussion with your doctor about your risks and potential benefits before deciding to have surgery (see Box 4-2, "Cataract surgery associated with reduced hip fractures").

Femtosecond laser

Pre-treating cataracts with a device called a femtosecond laser may result in safer, faster cataract surgery and better results, according to two studies presented at the annual meeting of the *American Academy of Ophthalmology*, October, 2011.

Standard cataract surgery via "phacoemulsification" begins with a tiny incision, followed by using ultrasound to emulsify the cataract for easy removal, and then insertion of an artificial intraocular lens. Outcomes are excellent in roughly 95 percent of healthy eyes. However, too much ultrasound can kill endothelial cells on the surface of the cornea. These cells are critical for clear vision, and they do not regenerate. Thus, conventional cataract surgery can result in vision that is no longer completely clear.

Laser treatment

Laser pretreatment of cataracts reduces the amount of ultrasound energy needed by nearly half. That eliminates loss of endothelial cells, according to the second of the two studies. Conversely, with standard treatment, cell loss ranges from one to seven percent. Refractive errors can be treated with the laser at the time of cataract surgery as well.

Earlier studies have revealed other benefits of femtosecond laser cataract surgery: Smaller incisions become possible, and improved removal of the lens capsule may reduce the likelihood of subsequent displacement of the artificial intraocular lens. This technique also seems to have improved results in patients who opt for advanced lenses that provide clear vision at any distance.

Many doctors recommend cataract surgery if your vision, with eyeglasses, is no better than 20/50, but that is not a hard-and-fast rule. The decision is yours to make based on how much the cataract interferes with your daily life. Can you see to read and do your work? Can you cook, clean and perform other basic daily activities? Do you feel comfortable driving? Is your impaired vision interfering with your independence? Or have you adjusted to the cataract, so that it doesn't interfere with your life? Insurance coverage also may factor into your decision to undergo cataract surgery. Medicare and most private health insurance policies will pay the costs of the cataract surgery, but you may have to pay extra for the so called "premium" intraocular lenses. Talk to your insurance company to find out how much of your surgical costs they will cover.

Eye complications

If you have other eye problems, such as diabetic retinopathy, your doctor may recommend that you have the cataract removed, even if it isn't causing vision problems, so that it doesn't interfere with the treatment of any other eye impairment. However, be aware that the risks of cataract surgery increase for people who have other diseases, particularly diabetes. Also, people with other eye conditions are less likely to see their vision improve following cataract surgery. The good news is that cataract surgery does not appear to speed the progression of age-related macular degeneration.

Living with cataracts

If you decide to put off surgery, you can often compensate for most, but not all of the vision loss associated with cataracts by using glasses. Talk to your doctor about scheduling regular eye exams to monitor your cataract. Ask your doctor to suggest low-vision aids or other methods to cope with the problem. You can also:

- Use a magnifying glass to help you read or do fine detail work.
- Update your eyeglass or contact lens prescription frequently.
- Limit night driving.
- Wear anti-glare sunglasses or yellow-tinted glasses to compensate for glare problems.

▶ **Improve the lighting in your home with stronger bulbs,** and position the light directly on your work, rather than shining it over your shoulder. Use lampshades and frosted bulbs to reduce glare.

Cataract surgery—what to expect

Cataract surgery works by removing the clouded lens and replacing it with a clear artificial lens. Before surgery, your doctor will give you some tests to measure the size and shape of your eye in order to implant the correct lens. If you have cataracts in both eyes, you will need two surgeries several months apart. Cataract surgery is never performed on both eyes on the same day.

Pre-op procedures

The night before surgery, do not eat or drink anything after midnight. If you normally take medications, you can do so with a small sip of water. However, be sure to inform your doctor about any medications you are taking, particularly tamsulosin (Flomax), a drug that is commonly used to treat an enlarged prostate, or blood thinners; these drugs may increase your risk of surgical complications. Your doctor may ask you to stop taking blood thinner medications temporarily. Usually, you are not asked to stop the alpha-blocker medications such as tamsulosin but the surgeon will want to know you take it since he or she will watch for certain complications, which in some cases are avoidable.

Once you're at the hospital, your eye will be washed and you'll get drops to dilate the pupil so your doctor has better access to the lens. Most people choose to stay awake during cataract surgery with just eye drops or an anesthetic injection to numb the eye, but you can opt for general anesthesia and be asleep throughout the surgery. The procedure is usually done in less than an hour, and most patients go home the same day. Outpatient cataract surgery appears to be just as safe and effective as staying overnight (which is rarely approved or covered by insurance), and it does not seem to increase the risk of post-operative complications. The doctor will usually perform one of two kinds of procedures, described below, both of which have similar outcomes.

Phacoemulsification

The most common form of cataract surgery is called phacoemulsification (see Box 4-3, "Phacoemulsification"). It uses the smallest incision, and therefore has the shortest recovery time.

If your doctor chooses phacoemulsification she or he will make a tiny incision, about ⅛ of an inch long, in the side of the cornea. The surgeon will insert a tiny probe that vibrates with ultrasound waves to break up the cataract. Then she or he will suction out the debris, leaving most of the outer capsule of the lens in place so that it can support the artificial lens. Finally, the doctor will implant the artificial lens—a folded-up bit of plastic, acrylic, or silicone that unfolds once it's in place. This new lens becomes a permanent part of your eye. Most people don't require a suture because the incision is so small. Healing should be quick, and you should notice an improvement in your vision within a few days.

Extracapsular cataract extraction

When a cataract has grown too large to be broken up with ultrasound waves, the doctor will do a procedure called extracapsular cataract extraction (see Box 4-4, "Extracapsular cataract extraction," on the following page). Used less frequently than phacoemulsification, extracapsular surgery involves making an incision about ⅜ of an inch wide in the cornea, through which the main part of the cataract

PHACOEMULSIFICATION   BOX 4-3

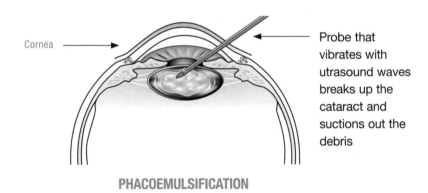

Cornea

Probe that vibrates with utrasound waves breaks up the cataract and suctions out the debris

PHACOEMULSIFICATION

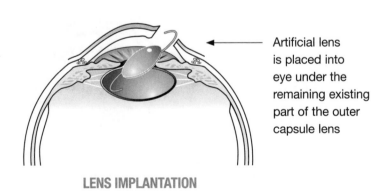

Artificial lens is placed into eye under the remaining existing part of the outer capsule lens

LENS IMPLANTATION

is surgically removed in one piece. The doctor then suctions out the rest of the lens, implants the artificial lens, and closes the incision with stitches. Because of the larger incision, healing after this procedure can take several weeks.

In rare cases, patients can't tolerate the artificial lens, called an intraocular lens, because of inflammation or other eye conditions. If this is the case with you, the doctor may remove the lens surgically without inserting a replacement intraocular lens. Instead, you will be fitted with special contact lenses or glasses to correct your vision. But sometimes such problems can be managed by removing one artificial intraocular lens and implanting another.

EXTRACAPSULAR CATARACT EXTRACTION

BOX 4-4

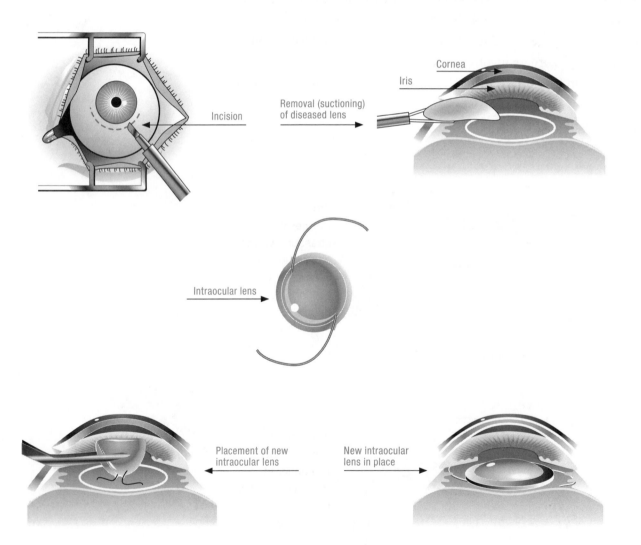

Incision

Removal (suctioning) of diseased lens

Cornea

Iris

Intraocular lens

Placement of new intraocular lens

New intraocular lens in place

After cataract surgery

After surgery, your eyes may itch and hurt and give off a pinkish-clear liquid discharge. They may also be very sensitive to light or touch. Your doctor can prescribe medications for the pain, which should clear up in a few days. You will be given antibiotic eye drops to prevent infection. You will need to wear an eye patch or glasses to protect your eye, and you should avoid rubbing it.

Post-op expectations

You should be able to resume normal activities soon after cataract surgery, but your vision may be blurry for a while during the healing period. You may also notice that colors appear much brighter now, because previously the cataract may have tinted your vision. You'll adjust to this change in time.

The implanted lens may give you 20/20 vision without glasses, but you may need a new eyeglass prescription after your eye has healed, because an unevenly shaped cornea after the surgery can cause astigmatism. In the past, most people had to wear reading glasses after cataract surgery. However, thanks to recent improvements in intraocular lenses, many people are now able to skip the reading glasses.

Accommodating and multifocal intraocular lenses are now available, which provide both near and distance vision. These lenses are flexible enough to mimic the younger eye's ability to focus on near and far objects. Patients appear to have high (as much as 90 percent) levels of satisfaction with implanted multifocal lenses, although a small percentage of patients have reported problems with glare and a halo effect around lights. A new variation of these lenses called the "dual optic" accommodating intraocular lens may improve visual contrast in low light compared to older multifocal lenses.

Revision surgery

Sometimes after surgery the remaining capsule of the natural lens that is left behind to support the artificial lens begins to cloud and obscure vision. This can happen months or even years later, in about 15 to 20 percent of patients. Often mistakenly called "after-cataract" or "secondary cataract," this clouding of the posterior capsule occurs when cells grow on the back of the lens capsule and obscure vision. It is easily treated with a laser procedure performed in less than five minutes in a doctor's office. A laser is used to cut a hole in the clouded portion of the lens capsule to let light through. You will have to stay in the doctor's office for about an hour after the procedure to be monitored for possible complications. The risks include elevated eye pressure (especially in people with glaucoma), swelling of the retina or, in rare cases, a detached retina, which can happen days, weeks, or even years after the procedure.

New developments

Researchers continue to look for better ways to prevent and treat cataracts. Many new intraocular lenses are under development. Focusing lenses are available, although they all have compromises. Additionally, the first lens that corrects high levels of astigmatism, the AcrySof® toric intraocular lens implant, was approved by the U.S. Food and Drug Administration in 2011. Also, surgeons are fine-tuning their techniques in the hope of reducing risks and shortening recovery time. In the future, lasers similar to the ones used for LASIK may replace manual incisions and phacoemulsification in cataract surgery. Researchers say these lasers, which are called femtosecond-pulse lasers, improve precision and safety, although they are more expensive than current surgical techniques.

5
GLAUCOMA

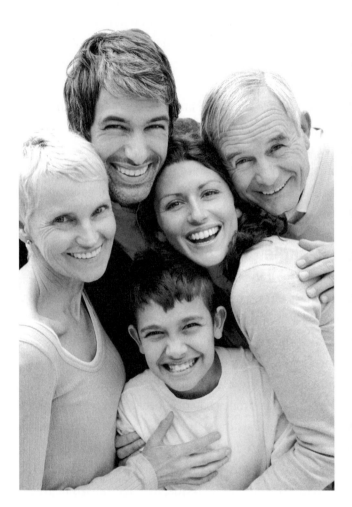
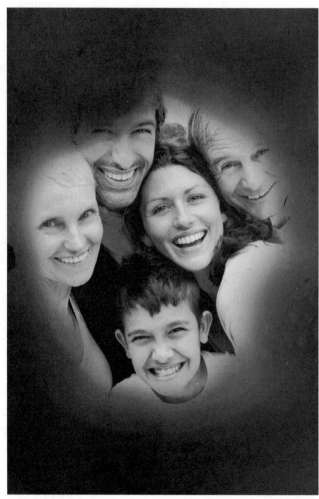

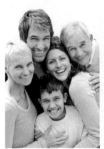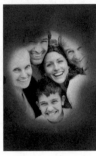

Normal vision   Vision with glaucoma

Glaucoma: No warning signs

Glaucoma is the number two cause of blindness in the world, second only to cataracts. It is also the leading cause of irreversible blindness in the world. In the U.S. alone, an estimated 2 million people have the disease, and an equal number of people likely have the disease but don't know it. By 2020, the disease is expected to have blinded more than 11 million people worldwide, according to the Glaucoma Research Foundation.

Because there are no symptoms until the disease is very advanced, glaucoma is a sneaky vision thief (see Box 5-1, "Normal vision vs. vision with glaucoma"). A National Eye Institute report found that fewer than 10 percent of Americans surveyed even knew that glaucoma had no warning signs. Once vision is lost to glaucoma, it's gone for good.

However, treatments have improved and now carry fewer side effects than in the past. Because doctors can usually control glaucoma once it's detected, stopping or at least slowing its progression to blindness, it's important to seek treatment soon after you've been diagnosed, and to be vigilant about taking medications to preserve your vision.

Primary open-angle glaucoma

The most common form of the disease, the one associated with aging, is called primary open-angle glaucoma. It's believed by many to be caused by problems in the trabecular meshwork, the fine meshwork that drains the aqueous humor from the eye, which is housed in the 'open angle' where the iris and cornea meet. Normally, the aqueous humor drains from the eye through this meshwork. That drainage maintains the proper balance, because the ciliary body constantly makes new fluid. But in open-angle glaucoma, the fluid does not drain quickly enough, leading to a surplus in the eye.

Researchers aren't sure why the drainage system malfunctions. It may be caused by natural aging of the tissue, damage caused by free radicals, genetics or other factors.

Whatever the cause, as the fluid builds up, the eye pressure rises (see Box 5-2, "Fluid build-up"). As pressure in the eye increases, it slowly damages the optic nerve. More and more optic nerve cells die off until vision begins to fade. First to go is the peripheral vision. Then the damage moves inward, eroding central vision until the person eventually goes blind.

Changes associated with glaucoma actually begin in the brain, damaging the axons—the ends of nerves—preventing the nerves from communicating with one-another. That damage eventually spreads to the optic nerve and retina. Researchers are currently looking for ways to restore those connections to help slow, or even prevent glaucoma.

Other research indicates that chemical changes inside the eye and optic nerve may spur the death of cells. This finding might lead to a new treatment approach that focuses on protecting the optic nerve from damage. For the time being, the only treatments proven to work are those that lower the pressure in the eye.

Though high eye pressure is a risk factor and often an early warning sign of glaucoma, it doesn't necessarily mean that nerve damage is occurring. Some people with high eye pressure never develop glaucoma. Others with normal pressure sustain nerve damage and are diagnosed with what is called low-tension or normal-tension glaucoma.

FLUID BUILD-UP BOX 5-2

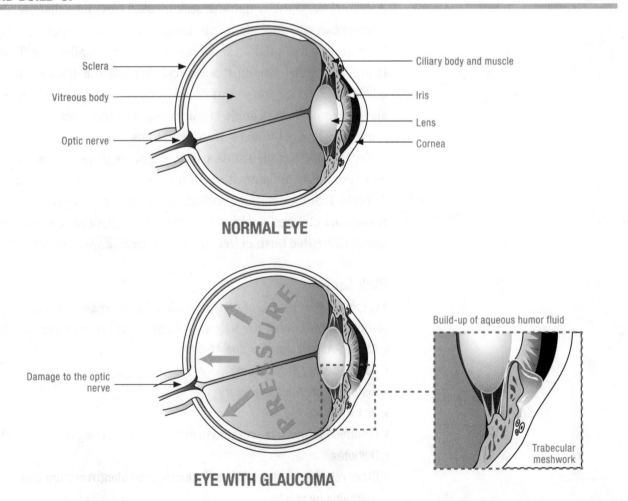

NORMAL EYE

EYE WITH GLAUCOMA

Angle-closure and other forms of glaucoma

There are other forms of glaucoma, as well. Some people are born with a malformation of the eye's drainage system, which puts them at risk for angle-closure glaucoma, a condition that occurs when the angle into which the aqueous fluid normally drains becomes completely blocked. Intermittently there is no drainage at all, and the eye pressure increases so rapidly that vision loss can progress to blindness within just one or two days if the situation is not treated aggressively. There are chronic forms of narrow angle glaucoma as well. Angle closure types of glaucoma are common in Asia.

Symptoms of angle-closure glaucoma include:
- Sudden blurry vision
- Severe eye pain
- Severe headache
- Colored halos forming around lights
- Nausea and vomiting
- Light sensitivity

If you have these symptoms, seek medical care immediately. Doctors can save your sight with prompt treatment, usually through laser surgery that pricks a small hole in your iris to allow the fluid to drain normally. You must act quickly because the disease acts quickly—and once you've lost vision, it can't be restored. There is also a chronic form of angle-closure glaucoma that does not lead to immediate loss of vision or acute symptoms.

Another form of glaucoma, called secondary glaucoma, is caused by an eye injury, inflammation, or infection, a very mature cataract, diabetes, lupus, or certain medications (particularly steroids). Sometimes children are born with congenital glaucoma, a rare and usually inherited birth defect that can be treated with surgery.

Risk factors

Everyone over the age of 60 is considered at increased risk for glaucoma, but any of the following factors increase risk even further:
- African-Americans over age 40
- Family history of glaucoma
- History of previous eye injury
- History of steroid use
- Elevated internal eye pressure (usually detected during an eye exam)
- Diabetes
- Other related health problems, including high blood pressure and migraine headaches

Having a family history of glaucoma has been linked to an increased risk. Studies of family members with glaucoma have helped researchers home in on potential genetic areas that may be involved in the disease. Researchers have identified a gene variant on chromosome 2 that they say dramatically increases an individual's risk for developing glaucoma. Mapping this and other genetic sites will help researchers develop new diagnostic tools and treatment methods for glaucoma (see Box 5-3, "Anti-convulsant topiramate may raise glaucoma risk").

Scientists have found an important connection between the genetic regions responsible for high blood pressure and glaucoma.

Blood pressure, thyroid issues are factors

High blood pressure is a risk factor for heart disease, which has also been linked to glaucoma. Research has found that people diagnosed with, or treated for open-angle glaucoma have a higher risk of death from heart disease, particularly if they have been treated with beta-blocker medication. More research is needed on this issue, but you should talk to your eye doctor if you have glaucoma and are on beta-blocker medications.

Having thyroid problems also might increase the risk for glaucoma. Excess sugar molecules (mucopolysaccharides), which can occur with underactive thyroid (hypothyroidism), can build up in the trabecular meshwork of the eye and raise intraocular pressure.

Prevention

Unfortunately, there is no proven way to prevent glaucoma completely. The best option is to get dilated eye exams and eye pressure checks every one to three years if you're between ages 55 and 64, and every one or two years after age 65, even if you have no symptoms of glaucoma. In some situations, if you have elevated eye pressure, even without glaucoma, research indicates that you can reduce your risk of glaucoma significantly by using the eye drops commonly prescribed to treat the disease. Starting treatment early helps delay or even prevents the disease in people at high risk for glaucoma, according to a recent study. Only 28 percent of those who started on medication at the beginning of the study developed primary open-angle glaucoma, compared to 40 percent of those who waited eight years before beginning medication treatment.

Even a small reduction in pressure can make a big difference in slowing vision loss. People with additional risk factors for glaucoma, such as those who are of African-American descent, are even more

NEW FINDING BOX 5-3

Anti-convulsant topiramate may raise glaucoma risk

Current use of the epilepsy drug, topiramate may be a slight risk factor for developing glaucoma, while new use of the drug may be a more substantial risk factor, according to a study in the May, 2012 *American Journal of Ophthalmology*. However, the drug did not appear to significantly worsen already existing cases of glaucoma. More studies are needed to confirm the findings, according to the report.

likely to benefit from treatment. If you have elevated eye pressure (greater than 20 mm Hg), talk to your doctor about your individual risks and how likely you are to benefit from treatment.

Prevention research
Better diagnostics

Using a model that looks at eye pressure and four other glaucoma risk factors, researchers are zeroing in on those at highest risk and pinpointing who might benefit most from preventive eye drops. The model is based on five criteria: age, intraocular pressure, appearance of the optic nerve head, corneal thickness, and the results of computerized visual field tests. Doctors can plug these five criteria into a Web-based calculator, and it will predict the chance a patient might develop glaucoma within five years. Although this model is still a work in progress, the researchers plan to fine-tune it as genetic and other risk factors for glaucoma emerge.

Impact of exercise

Some research has suggested that cardiovascular exercise can help reduce eye pressure. A study published in the October 2011 *Investigative Ophthalmology & Visual Science* showed that people with a long history of moderate exercise have a marker for a reduced risk of glaucoma. However, lifting heavy weights may not be the best option, because it may cause a temporary increase in eye pressure, especially when weight-lifters hold their breath during repetitions. (Forcing air against a closed windpipe tends to increase pressure inside the eyeball.)

Diet

Other researchers are investigating whether a diet high in fruits and vegetables, which contain antioxidants, may help ward off the disease, but that evidence is not conclusive at this time. (A diet high in fruit and vegetables generally promotes health, however, including some aspects of eye health.) The evidence on statin drugs, which lower cholesterol, is also promising. These drugs may decrease the likelihood of developing glaucoma, but so far there is not enough evidence to justify taking statins for glaucoma prevention, particularly because these drugs carry their own risk of side effects.

You may have heard about using marijuana to treat or prevent glaucoma. Research has found that marijuana actually does lower pressure in the eye temporarily, but the effect only works for a few hours. It would require smoking eight to 10 marijuana cigarettes around the clock to sustain the necessary drop in eye pressure.

Researchers believe this is impractical, and in most states, it is illegal. In their search for a more practical alternative, researchers have focused on compounds derived from marijuana, which they believe might lead to an effective—and legal—glaucoma drug.

Screening tools

You may be familiar with the "air puff" test used to screen for glaucoma. This test detects elevated eye pressure, which is an important risk factor, but by itself is not sufficient to diagnose the disease. The only true way to catch glaucoma early is with a full dilated-eye exam in which the doctor looks for signs of trouble with the optic nerve.

A comprehensive glaucoma screening may include one or more of the following tests:

• Tonometry: a more accurate test of internal eye pressure. The normal range is considered to be a score of between 12 and 21 mm Hg (although some types of glaucoma can occur with pressures below 21 mm Hg). The test may have to be repeated, as eye pressure can vary at different times of the day.

• Slit lamp and hand-held ophthalmoscope: an examination of the optic nerve to check for deterioration.

• Gonioscopy: using a special contact lens that contains mirrors to enable the doctor to see the angle that is causing the problem and to check the extent of blockage in the drainage area.

• Photography: computerized imaging of the optic nerve to assess damage.

• Visual field testing: checking your peripheral vision to see how badly your sight has been compromised. During this test, lights are flashed into your eyes to determine whether you can see them in your central and peripheral vision.

• Pachymetry: a technique that measures the thickness of your cornea might help assess your risk of developing glaucoma. People with thick corneas may have an artificially high pressure reading. Those with thin corneas can have normal pressure but still have glaucoma.

Other tests

In recent years, new tests to analyze the thickness of optic nerve fibers have emerged, including Heidelberg Retinal Tomography (HRT II) and optical coherence tomography (OCT). These tests create computerized images of the optic nerve to look for damage. Researchers are also investigating a test called PERGLA, which may be able to detect damage before it becomes irreversible, according to a recent study. It may also be worth testing patients with conditions such as

Peripheral vision loss from glaucoma may increase auto crash risk

Drivers with glaucoma had about twice as many crashes as those with healthy eyes, according to a Japanese study that used a driving simulator to compare the two groups. The research was presented at the 2012 annual meeting of the American Academy of Ophthalmology, in November.

Glaucoma can rob sufferers of peripheral vision, without affecting central vision including visual acuity, until late in the course of the disease. Driver's license exams in many states do not test peripheral vision. In the driving simulation study, the greatest number of crashes involved another vehicle or pedestrian crossing into a driver's path from the side. Under these circumstances, subjects with glaucoma were more than twice as likely to collide with the interloper.

high blood pressure, high cholesterol, lupus and diabetes for glaucoma, as patients with glaucoma are also at significantly higher risk for these health conditions.

Diagnosis

If you've been diagnosed with glaucoma, you will need to see your doctor regularly, and these tests will be repeated to determine whether treatment is working. Sometimes glaucoma treatments stop working after a while, and your doctor will want to try other options, so you must be vigilant about returning for frequent follow-up eye exams.

Treatment

There is no cure for glaucoma, but studies have shown that treatment to lower eye pressure can usually control the disease, reducing and delaying further vision loss.

Research has demonstrated that lowering eye pressure can prevent blindness in many patients, and it may delay the progression of vision difficulties. Keeping intraocular pressure at a steady low may help reduce the risk of sight loss. Fluctuations in eye pressure are thought to put undue stress on the eye tissues, leading to increased damage.

Typically, most glaucoma patients are started on eye drops first. In recent years, some doctors have begun treating their patients with laser surgery first (a practice that is more common in Europe) to reduce or avoid the need for drugs which may be inconvenient, may have side effects, and over time, may be more costly than laser surgery. You may want to discuss the pros and cons of this option with your eye doctor, as research has shown laser surgery to be safe and effective. Because drug treatments and surgery have improved greatly in recent years, changing medications or switching to laser surgery can be valid options for preserving vision. Discuss the risks and potential benefits of each treatment with your ophthalmologist before making a decision (see Box 5-4, "Peripheral vision loss from glaucoma may increase auto crash risk").

Medications

In the U.S., drugs are typically the first line of defense in treating glaucoma, and a variety of different classes and formulations have been developed, most of which are in the form of eye drops.

Eye drops

Some drops help fluid drain from the eye; others reduce the amount of fluid the eye produces. Before beginning a drug regimen for glaucoma, you should tell the ophthalmologist about your full medical history and any medications you are taking. Some drugs can interact with glaucoma medications and cause dangerous problems.

Also, talk to your eye doctor about your schedule and lifestyle so that the two of you can develop a treatment regimen you can sustain. For example, if certain drops interfere with your driving ability, you want to be sure they are timed not to interfere with your commute. Most people are able to tolerate glaucoma medication and do not experience side effects, but problems can occur. If you do have side effects, ask your ophthalmologist about changing your regimen or perhaps trying surgery as an alternative. Here's a look at your medication options:

▶ **Prostaglandins** improve the drainage of fluid from the eye, and they have the advantage of once-daily dosing. These drugs include Xalatan, Lumigan, Travatan, and Tafluprost. Among their side effects are blurred vision, allergic reactions, headache, and fatigue, as well as cosmetic changes to the eye—they can turn blue eyes brown and cause your lashes to grow longer and thicker. Tafluprost has some potentially serious side effects, including macular edema (swelling of the center of the retina). Newer prostaglandin drugs seem mostly to have fewer side effects than older medications.

▶ **Prostamides** increase the flow of fluid from the eye. Side effects include red or itchy eyes.

▶ **Beta-blockers** reduce the amount of aqueous humor the eye produces. Possible side effects are rare but can be serious. They include difficulty breathing, slowed heart rate and blood pressure, impotence, fatigue and depression. These drugs should be used with caution in patients who have breathing problems or heart disease.

▶ **Alpha-agonists** such as AlphaganP and iopidine reduce the amount of fluid produced and increase drainage from the eye. Side effects include irritation, dry mouth and fatigue.

▶ **Topical carbonic anhydrase inhibitors**, including Trusopt and Azopt, reduce the amount of fluid in the eye. In some cases, these drugs can cause burning and blurred vision. If the drops don't work for you, your doctor may prescribe oral carbonic anhydrase inhibitors in pill form—such as Diamox and Neptazane. These work as well as eye drops but, because the medicine travels throughout your body, pills are more likely to cause side effects such as numbness in the hands and feet, depression, anemia, lethargy and excessive urination.

▶ **Miotics** work by constricting the pupil and opening the eye's drainage system, allowing more fluid to pass from the eye. Side effects of this medication class include blurred vision, headache, extreme nearsightedness and problems with night vision.

- ► Adrenergics are almost never used anymore because they are less effective than newer drugs. They work by increasing drainage and reducing the amount of fluid produced in the eye. Adrenergics can cause red eye, heart palpitations, increased blood pressure, headaches and anxiety.
- ► Combination treatments may be more effective for some patients who need more than one drug, and they also may simplify the drug regimen. Combigan is a regimen that combines the alpha agonist, brimonidine, with the beta-blocker, timolol. Cosopt combines a beta-blocker with a carbonic anhydrase inhibitor.

Research has found that four medications—bimatoprost (Lumigan), travoprost (Travatan), latanoprost (Xalatan) and timolol (Timoptic)—seem to do a better job of lowering eye pressure than other available drugs. However, certain risk factors and responses to drugs can cause results to vary. You will need to work with your doctor to find a drug regimen that works for you.

Stents lower pressure

A potential new treatment option is the use of tiny drains the size of an eyelash, called stents, which during a clinical trial lowered intraocular pressure so stably that after six months, patients were able to dispense with eyedrops (see Box 5-5, "Insertion of tiny drains may improve control of intraocular pressure"). These mini-stents could also be used for open-angle glaucoma earlier in the course of the disease than other medications, and with fewer complications.

Under development

Several new medications are in development. Researchers are reviewing an experimental drug that could slow the progression of glaucoma and delay sight loss in a new way. The drug, called memantine, is already being used to treat Parkinson's and Alzheimer's diseases. With glaucoma, it works by preventing the build-up of nerve-damaging calcium in the optic nerve. If it proves effective, memantine would be the first oral medication for glaucoma that directly protects the optic nerve.

Azheimer's-glaucoma link

Scientists are investigating other treatment options based on the relationship between glaucoma and Alzheimer's disease. They have found that amyloid-b peptide, the substance that forms harmful plaques in the brains of people with Alzheimer's, also kills retina cells in rat models of glaucoma. By targeting this substance with medication, they hope to slow the progression of glaucoma. Combining three drugs that prevent amyloid-b buildup works very well at preventing cell death in the retina.

Follow your regimen

Because glaucoma is painless and has so few symptoms in its early stages, many people stop their medications due to neglect, denial, cost, complicated regimens or side effects. If you're not consistent with your regimen, you could increase your risk of future vision loss. Here are some strategies for creating a medication regimen you can stick with:

▸ **Ask your doctor to fully explain your treatment plan,** including your drug dosing schedule, and potential side effects. Be sure to keep asking questions until you're comfortable with your regimen.

▸ **Ask your doctor to simplify your treatment plan as much as possible.** Taking the smallest dosage possible the fewest number of times per day can minimize side effects and make it easier for you to stay on schedule.

▸ **Talk to your doctor about adjusting your treatment schedule to fit your lifestyle.** You'll be much more likely to take your medication if it doesn't interfere with your daily routine.

NEW FINDING BOX 5-5

Insertion of tiny drains may improve control of intraocular pressure

A major challenge in treating glaucoma is to maintain reduced intraocular pressure, a task which requires consistent and regular use of pressure lowering medicines by patients. Sustained release medications and/or drainage devices may improve convenience, resulting in better control and better results.

A tiny drain, or "stent" the size of an eyelash, which is implanted during minimally invasive surgery or during cataract surgery, as part of a clinical trial, decreased intraocular pressure stably. At six months out, most patients no longer needed eye drop medications, according to research presented at the 116th Annual Meeting of the American Academy of Ophthalmology, November 2012.

Tiny stents enable treatment of open-angle glaucoma sooner in the disease process, and with lower complication rates, Thomas W. Samuelson, M.D., the medical monitor for the clinical trial said at the annual meeting. No significant complications were detected during the clinical trial. "If the devices can effectively control [intraocular pressure] over many years, it would be a real breakthrough in combating this blinding disease," said Samuelson.

Current treatment choices have shortcomings. Some patients fail to apply their eye drops consistently enough to control the disease; others simply do not respond well to drugs. Current surgical procedures for opening blocked drainage channels or implanting larger stents, which are used only in cases of advanced glaucoma, carry risks of substantial complications, including vision loss.

Other mini-stents are being developed, and some are in clinical trials. One, the iStent, has been approved by the US Food and Drug Administration. It must be implanted during cataract surgery.

Several more years will be necessary to determine long-term safety and efficacy with the new mini-stents.

- Keep a schedule of your doses, or buy a pill box that can help you organize your medications for the day. Eye drop bottles may fit in some of these "organizers." If vision impairment makes it difficult for you to write, have someone create a schedule for you, using big letters you can see—or use colored stickers to indicate which medications you need to take at what times.
- Don't be shy about voicing cost concerns. Your doctor may be able to substitute a less costly drug or direct you to payment assistance plans.
- Follow your doctor's instructions carefully when using your eye drops. Taking eye drops correctly is important, both to ensure that your treatment plan works and to reduce side effects. Here are some tips:
    1. Always wash your hands before touching the bottle or your eye.
    2. Tilt your head back and hold the bottle as close as you can to your eye without touching it.
    3. With your free hand, pull down your lower eyelid to form a little bowl.
    4. Place the correct number of drops into the bowl. If you need more than one kind of drop, wait five minutes before taking the next set.
    5. Close your eyes and press your finger against your lower lid near your nose. This is important to prevent the drops from draining away into your tear ducts, which can increase the risk of side effects and decrease the drops' effectiveness.

Surgery

If your medications don't work, your doctor may advise surgery. You have two options: laser surgery or conventional surgery. Typically, patients are offered laser surgery first. Before you decide on surgery, you should discuss your full medical history with your ophthalmologist, to assess your risk of side effects and prospects for success.

Laser surgery

Laser surgery works by burning holes into the meshwork of tissue in the angle of the eye to allow more fluid to drain. Surgery may be more effective than medication for controlling intraocular pressure in glaucoma patients with advanced disease who are taking the maximum amount of medication.

Trabeculoplasty

Trabeculoplasty is a type of laser surgery that is performed as an outpatient procedure in a doctor's office in 10-20 minutes. If you elect to have this procedure, you will receive drops to numb your eye. The doctor will use a high-energy laser to burn holes in the drainage canals and allow the fluid to drain more easily. Following the procedure, your doctor will want to recheck your internal eye pressure several times. You will receive medications to control inflammation, as well as regular glaucoma drugs. You may have some blurred vision, inflammation and sensitivity to light after the operation, but these problems are usually temporary.

Conventional surgery

Some patients don't respond well to laser surgery. For most people, surgery is not a permanent solution. More than half of patients later require conventional surgery because their eye pressure rises within two years after a laser procedure. Because the laser procedure carries less risk than conventional surgery, however, many doctors advise trying it first. You should also be aware that the surgery may not eliminate the need for drugs. More than half of all patients experience worsening eye pressure after surgery, and eventually require more drugs. However, having surgery may allow you to reduce your dosage or delay taking certain medications.

Selective laser trabeculoplasty

A relatively new version of laser surgery is called selective laser trabeculoplasty (SLT) (see Box 5-6, "Selective laser trabeculoplasty").

SELECTIVE LASER TRABECULOPLASTY   BOX 5-6

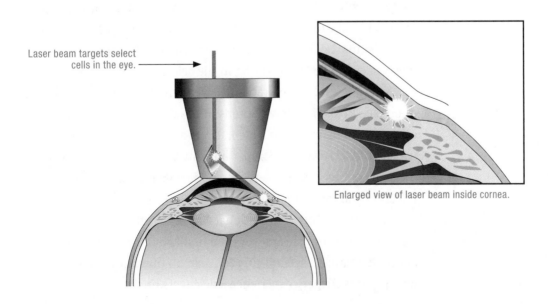

Laser beam targets select cells in the eye.

Enlarged view of laser beam inside cornea.

It differs from conventional laser surgery in that it uses a laser to target only selected cells in the eye. For this reason, it causes less tissue damage than conventional laser surgery, while still improving the drainage of fluid from the eye. SLT can be performed on an outpatient basis.

Research is showing that this procedure reduces intraocular pressure by about 30 percent. Patients appear to maintain that lower pressure for as long as five years. Advocates of this surgery hope that it will lessen the need for conventional surgery and perhaps even reduce or replace medications as a first-line treatment for glaucoma. However, randomized controlled trials comparing SLT with traditional laser trabeculoplasty and medication will need to be done to confirm its effectiveness.

Surgery of last resort

Conventional surgery is usually offered to patients when medications and laser surgery have failed, if there is significant damage to an untreated eye or if there is scarring. It works by creating a new alternative drainage system to replace the natural meshwork drain. Sometimes, doctors need to implant a tiny plastic valve into a new drainage hole to ensure that it stays open to drain properly, or they use a laser to kill most of the cells in the ciliary body that produce the aqueous humor. This procedure is considered risky and is often reserved as a last resort for patients who haven't responded to other treatments.

Outpatient surgery

Surgery is usually performed on an outpatient basis at a hospital or surgery center. The anesthesiologist will give you medications to relax you and will inject drugs to numb your eye before the operation. The most common procedure is called a trabeculectomy, and it involves cutting a tiny opening in the sclera, the white part of the eye. This allows fluid to drain out, bypassing the clogged meshwork drain (see Box 5-7, "Flow of fluids in the eye post-surgery"). Typically, a tiny blister, called a bleb, forms over the incision, but it is usually hidden under the upper lid. You should be able to go home the same day as your surgery. You will be given drops to prevent infection and inflammation.

For most patients, conventional surgery is effective and long lasting, but it does not always work the first time. About 40 percent of people require a second surgery. A small number of people who undergo this surgery experience side effects, including infection, problems with the cornea, bleeding, drooping eyelid, fluid accumulation within the eye walls, retinal detachment or cataracts. Some patients will see shadows due to a buildup of fluid in the back of the eye. In rare cases, the surgery can worsen vision or even lead to blindness.

This is a promising time for glaucoma patients. New drugs are under investigation that should reduce side effects and improve the treatment success rate. Other areas of research that may someday offer hope are focused on regenerating the optic nerve. A number of genes involved in glaucoma have been identified, giving researchers promising targets for new drugs and therapies, and perhaps a way to spot those most at risk for the disease.

FLOW OF FLUIDS IN THE EYE POST-SURGERY   BOX 5-7

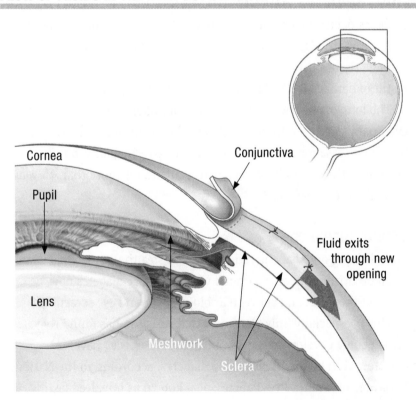

Cornea

Conjunctiva

Pupil

Fluid exits through new opening

Lens

Meshwork

Sclera

Diabetic retinopathy afflicts
approximately 4.2 million
people who have diabetes.

6 DIABETIC RETINOPATHY

Diabetic retinopathy, a complication of diabetes, is the leading cause of new blindness in people between the ages of 20 and 74. It develops when diabetes damages the blood vessels that feed the retina. Diabetic retinopathy afflicts approximately 4.2 million people who have diabetes. That means nearly a third of all people with diabetes have diabetic retinopathy, according to the National Institute of Diabetes and Digestive and Kidney Diseases (NIDDK). In more than 4 percent of these people, the condition is severe enough to threaten their sight. The number of people with diabetic retinopathy is expected to increase dramatically in the coming decades. That's because the population is aging, and growing more obese, two phenomena which lead to a rapidly rising rate of diabetes. Experts predict that 16 million Americans will have diabetic retinopathy by the year 2050, and 3.4 million of these will be at risk of losing their sight from the disease. Diabetes patients are also at increased risk for cataracts, glaucoma and several other vision problems, which is why tight control of blood sugar and regular vision screening are so important.

How diabetes affects the eye

Diabetes occurs when your body is unable to break down and process sugar properly. This causes blood sugar levels to rise, which can damage tissues throughout your body. Diabetic retinopathy is the result of damage to the blood vessels that feed the retina.

The longer you have diabetes, the more likely it is that you will eventually develop retinopathy. Only 10 percent of people who have had the disease for less than five years have retinopathy, but 70 percent of those who have lived with diabetes for more than 15 years have this eye disease.

Stealth diseases

Both diabetes and diabetic retinopathy are stealth diseases that can creep up unannounced. So even if you don't have diabetes now, be aware of the risks, and get regular blood sugar and eye screenings.

This is especially important now that research has found that some people develop diabetic retinopathy when they have pre-diabetes, even before they develop diabetes, according to the National Institutes of Health. Pre-diabetes, also known as impaired fasting glucose, or impaired glucose tolerance, is a condition in which people have higher-than-normal blood glucose levels that aren't yet high enough to qualify for an official diagnosis of diabetes. (A new study shows that the prevalence of non-refractive visual impairment, generally, has risen in tandem with diabetes (see Box 6-1, "Link between rise in diabetes and non-refractive visual impairment"). Pre-diabetes can lead to diabetes, but with proper weight control and nutrition, many people can prevent the progression.

If you have diabetes, don't skip your annual dilated eye exam. Diabetic retinopathy can be treated successfully more than 95 percent of the time if caught early, but it can cause blindness if detected late and left untreated.

The American Academy of Ophthalmology recommends this screening schedule for all diabetes patients:

▶ **If you are diagnosed with diabetes before age 30,** your first comprehensive eye exam should be five years later, or at age 10, whichever is later.

▶ **If you are diagnosed after age 30,** you should have a comprehensive eye exam at the time of diagnosis.

Once you've had your initial eye exam, you should have a follow-up examination at least once every year, unless you have another eye condition or levels of retinopathy that require more frequent attention.

Two basic types of diabetic retinopathy
Nonproliferative diabetic retinopathy

Nonproliferative diabetic retinopathy is the early stage of the disease. It starts when the walls of the blood vessels in the retina weaken, causing tiny bulges in the blood vessels. These bulges, called microaneurysms, may then leak blood and fluid into the retina. The presence of outpouchings indicates the mild stage of diabetic retinopathy. When some of the blood vessels start to become blocked, the disease has progressed to moderate nonproliferative retinopathy. In the final, severe stage, many more blood vessels are blocked, and parts of the retina lose their blood supply.

The mild stage of diabetic retinopathy may not affect your vision, but as the blood vessels weaken and leak more fluid, they can cause your macula to swell in a condition called macular edema. Though more common in the later stages of diabetic retinopathy, macular edema can develop early and lead to blurring of your central vision. If the macula loses its blood supply, your central vision will decline.

Proliferative diabetic retinopathy

Eventually, when many blood vessels are blocked and the retina is starving from a lack of nutrient-carrying blood, new blood vessels begin to grow on the retinal surface and into the vitreous in an attempt to bring blood to the retina. This is the more severe stage of retinopathy, called **proliferative diabetic retinopathy**. Up to 75 percent of people with severe nonproliferative diabetic retinopathy will progress to the vision-threatening proliferative form within one year (see Box 6-2, "Proliferative diabetic retinopathy").

With this form of the disease, the new blood vessels that rush to rescue the retina are abnormal, fragile and susceptible to leaking. Because they can grow on the retina and other eye structures, if they bleed or scar they can dramatically affect both central and peripheral vision, leading to retinal detachment. They also can bleed into the vitreous gel ("vitreous hemorrhage"), clouding or even blocking vision. Sometimes scar tissue forms as the blood vessels contract. This can pull the retina off the back wall of the eye, which can cause serious vision loss and even permanent blindness. Sometimes, blood vessels grow onto the iris and block the eye's drainage system, causing a dangerous form of glaucoma called neovascular glaucoma.

PROLIFERATIVE DIABETIC RETINOPATHY BOX 6-2

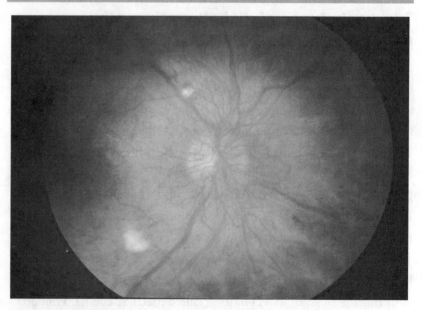

Proliferative diabetic retinopathy is the later stage of the disease that occurs when new, abnormal blood vessels begin to grow on the surface of the retina and into the vitreous humor. Note the interconnected, lacy, thin, filigree-like new blood vessels that form a network over the optic nerve head.

Risk factors

Everyone with diabetes is at risk of developing diabetic retinopathy. Your risk increases the longer you have diabetes and the less control you have over your blood sugar. High blood sugar levels presumably damage the retina over time. People who have type 1 diabetes, which tends to start early in life, are at higher risk for retinopathy partly because they may have had diabetes for longer. But people with type 2 diabetes, formerly known as adult-onset diabetes, are also at risk. This disease can occur even in patients whose blood sugar levels are below the 7.0 millimoles/liter (mmol/L) threshold normally used to diagnose diabetes. For this reason, researchers have suggested that doctors combine other diabetes risk factors with blood sugar levels to determine a person's risk for diabetic retinopathy. These risk factors include:

- High blood pressure
- High hemoglobin A1c (a measure of blood sugar control)
- Obesity
- High cholesterol levels
- Kidney problems
- Infections

Prevention

The most important thing you can do to prevent diabetic retinopathy is to **keep tight control of your blood sugar**. Watching your blood pressure will also reduce your risk. One study found that people with diabetic retinopathy who control their blood pressure with medication are 25 percent less likely to go blind.

Other things you can do to reduce your risk include:

- **Don't smoke.** Smoking shuts down blood vessels and may worsen retinopathy.
- **Lower your cholesterol and lipid levels.**
- **Be alert for vision changes.** If you are between regular eye exams and notice vision changes that last for more than a few days, or are not associated with a change in blood sugar, see an ophthalmologist as soon as possible.

Symptoms

The early stages of diabetic retinopathy often produce no symptoms. What's more, some people with diabetes ignore blurry vision because they know that high blood sugar levels can temporarily blur vision. The blurred vision caused by macular edema may change over the course of the day, growing better or worse as the swelling ebbs and flows, but it will usually not improve without treatment. Also, if new blood vessels are bleeding, you may notice spots floating in your field of vision. If in doubt, have a doctor examine your eyes.

Because diabetic retinopathy can progress to an advanced and less treatable stage without causing symptoms or pain, it's important to get an annual dilated eye exam, as well as to have any follow-ups your ophthalmologist thinks are necessary. The exam can also catch glaucoma and cataracts, which diabetics are at a higher risk of developing.

Here are some symptoms that should send you to your ophthalmologist's office immediately for an examination:

- Spots or "cobwebs" floating in your vision
- Dark streaks or a red haze that blocks vision
- Vision loss, sometimes in both eyes, but usually in just one eye
- Blurred vision
- A blind spot in the center of your vision
- Poor night vision
- Difficulty adjusting to changes in light

If you see many new floaters, it is possible that new blood vessels have begun to bleed and you should see your doctor as soon as possible, even if these floaters clear up on their own. Once bleeding occurs, it is likely to return and it may get progressively worse, causing serious vision loss or even blindness. The earlier you seek treatment, the more likely that treatment is to succeed.

Diagnosis

It's important for diabetes patients to get regular eye exams, yet studies show only 50 to 70 percent get the recommended annual eye check-ups. Your doctor will do a dilated eye exam to assess your level of diabetic retinopathy and determine whether you require treatment. He or she will use the slit lamp to check your retina for signs of damage. Your doctor may also suggest a fluorescein angiogram or an optical coherence tomography (OCT) scan to determine the extent and location of any leakage or bleeding, and to help plan your treatment. The angiogram involves injecting a fluorescent dye into your arm and then taking pictures as the dye passes through the blood vessels in your retina.

There are a small number of "telemedicine" screening options available in some areas. For example, a new device, Retasure, diagnoses diabetic retinopathy by taking digital photographs of the retina, and then transmitting the images to a board-certified ophthalmologist, who checks for signs of the disease. Another new test on the horizon might be even more accurate than standard vision tests for picking up subtle sight loss, and it could help doctors determine whether diabetic retinopathy treatments are working. This technique, called **flavoprotein autofluorescence**, detects proteins that turn fluorescent during times of metabolic stress, which often occurs in the early stages of the disease before symptoms appear.

Treatment

The most important thing you can do—before retinopathy is diagnosed and also in its early stages—is to **maintain tight control over your blood sugar levels, blood pressure and serum lipids, or cholesterol**. Diabetics who tightly control their blood sugar can significantly reduce their risk of developing diabetic retinopathy, and if they already have the condition, can reduce their risk of the disease progressing.

Good control, which has been shown to greatly lower the risk of all diabetic complications, requires you to monitor your blood sugar levels closely and use insulin or other hypoglycemic drugs as needed to keep your blood sugar at levels similar to those in non-diabetics. You will have to work with your general physician or endocrinologist to develop a plan for control. It's also a good idea to take a diabetes education class.

Cardiac complications from certain drugs

In the past, one way to control blood sugar levels was with medications such as rosiglitazone (Avandia). Research suggests that taking this drug can reduce the risk of diabetic retinopathy by almost 60 percent. However, Avandia and other drugs in its class may actually increase the risk of developing the more serious diabetic macular edema, and are now under review for their potential role in cardiovascular risk. Two recent studies reported that Avandia caused cardiovascular complications, including heart attack, stroke and congestive heart failure in people over age 65 with diabetes. In September 2010, the European Union suspended all sales of the rosiglitazone-containing medicines—Avandia, Avandamet, and Avaglim. In 2011, the U.S. Food and Drug Administration limited the use of rosiglitazone medications, including Avandia, to healthcare providers and patients enrolled in a special access program. Avandia is no longer available through retail pharmacies. Pioglitazone (Actos), a drug that activates a similar mechanism in the body, does not seem to increase risk of cardiovascular events. However, that drug also is undergoing FDA scrutiny for possible side effects.

Tried and true treatment

One way to combat macular edema appears to be with the same medications used to treat age-related macular degeneration. In two

Lucentis approved for diabetic macular edema

The US Food and Drug Administration approved Lucentis for diabetic macular edema, in August, 2012. Diabetic macular edema—a swelling of the central retina—is a complication of types 1 and 2 diabetes, which can cause blindness in severe cases.

Lucentis had been previously approved for neovascular, or wet age-related macular degeneration, and for macular edema due to retinal vein occlusion.

The approval specifies that the drug should be given monthly, by injection into the vitreous cavity of the eyeball. Additional studies have shown that Lucentis may also be combined with laser treatment for diabetic macular edema.

BOX 6-4

Type 2 diabetes drug effective against diabetic retinopathy

The use of fenofibrate as an adjunctive treatment for diabetic retinopathy is now supported by strong clinical data, according to a paper in the July, 2012 *American Journal of Ophthalmology*. Fenofibrate reduced progression of diabetic retinopathy by 30%-40% over four to five years, according to the report. Patients with preexisting retinopathy at the start of the trial received greater benefit than those without.

Since eye doctors neither prescribe, nor typically consider which diabetes medications their patients should take, this is an issue patients should discuss with their primary care doctor, or any other doctor who is prescribing their diabetes medications.

The paper was a review of two trials, and included 11,388 patients with type 2 diabetes, who had taken fenofibrate for as long as five years.

sets of clinical trials published together in the April 2012 *Ophthalmology*, Lucentis was shown to boost vision for diabetic macular edema patients by at least three lines on the Snellen Eye Chart, for nearly half of the subjects receiving the drug. These improvements occurred quickly, and endured over the entire course of the two-year trials. Other studies, such as one conducted by the Diabetic Retinopathy Clinical Research Network study group have shown that combining Lucentis with laser treatment for patients with diabetic macular edema improves outcomes compared to laser treatment alone (see Box 6-3, "Lucentis approved for diabetic macular edema").

Avastin, like Lucentis, also can stabilize, or even improve, vision in diabetes patients with macular edema. This treatment is now being used together with laser treatment to manage many patients with diabetic macular edema, and in some cases Avastin or Lucentis (or in the future, other drugs such as Eylea) may eventually replace laser photocoagulation for macular edema.

Controlling risk factors with drugs

Keeping other risk factors, such as blood pressure, under control can also help preserve your sight. Candesartan (Atacand)—a drug used to treat high blood pressure—appears to be effective at preventing and treating diabetic retinopathy. Two other high blood pressure medications—losartan (Cozar) and enalapril (Vasotec)—can slow the progression of retinopathy by 60 to 70 percent in patients with type 1 diabetes. Although these results are promising, more research needs to be done to determine which patients are most likely to benefit from this therapy, and for how long therapy should be given.

A new study, published in the July, 2012 *American Journal of Ophthalmology* showed that Fenofibrate used as an adjunctive treatment slowed the progression of diabetic retinopathy quite significantly (see Box 6-4, "Type 2 diabetes drug effective against diabetic retinopathy"). However, the systemic management of diabetes mellitus is complex and should be discussed with the patient's endocrinologist or primary care doctor managing the diabetes.

Controlling your diabetes reduces your long-term risk of retinopathy, but in the short term it can actually worsen retinopathy in a small percentage of patients, particularly in those who have had poor control of their blood sugar for a long time. Remember, too, that while tight control greatly reduces your risk of retinopathy and severe vision loss, it doesn't eliminate it.

However, researchers have found that good control is still beneficial, because after a few years even patients whose condition worsens are better off than if they had not controlled their blood sugar. If you are starting a blood sugar control program, discuss your risks with the doctor who normally treats your diabetes. Researchers have suggested that patients at risk for early worsening should have dilated eye exams at least once every three months for the first six months to a year after starting the tight control program.

If your retinopathy does progress, your doctor will want to monitor your eyes frequently. There are several treatments available to prevent and control vision loss.

Laser surgery (photocoagulation)

The most common treatment is laser surgery (**photocoagulation**) to stop the leakage and growth of new blood vessels. Research finds this treatment can reduce the risk of severe vision loss by 50 percent. Photocoagulation uses a laser to burn parts of the retinal blood vessels that have abnormal outpouchings, to seal any leaks. You'll probably have this surgery in your doctor's office or at a surgery center on an outpatient basis.

The doctor will give you drops to dilate the pupils and numb your eyes. You may also need shots around the eye to prevent pain. Your doctor will place a special contact lens on your cornea to focus the laser onto the correct areas of your retina. During the procedure you may see bright flashes of light, which may produce a stinging sensation.

Macular edema

If you are being treated for **macular edema**, the laser will seal leaking blood vessels around the macula. This may take up to several hundred tiny laser burns. Called focal laser treatment, this procedure can reduce the risk of vision loss by 50 percent, and it often stabilizes vision (see Box 6-5, "Focal laser treatment," on the following page). On rare occasions, it may even improve vision.

Proliferative retinopathy

If you have **proliferative retinopathy**, the laser will be focused on the peripheral retina, avoiding the macula. Your doctor may make up to 1500-2,000 laser burns over one or several sessions (see Box 6-6, "Scatter laser treatment"). These burns shrink the abnormal blood vessels, though exactly how they work isn't completely understood. The surgery, which is called scatter laser treatment or panretinal photocoagulation, can cause some loss of your peripheral and night vision. It also may slightly reduce your color vision and cause some temporary blurring of your central vision, but it can save the rest of your sight and prevent blindness. Scatter laser treatment works better before the abnormal blood vessels have started to bleed, though it is still feasible if the bleeding isn't yet too severe.

Post-op effects

After both types of laser surgery, it will probably be advisable to have someone drive you home. Your eyes will remain dilated for a while, so you'll need to wear sunglasses. You may have temporarily blurred vision and some eye pain or a headache. You may see some small spots after laser treatment, but they usually fade away over time. Bleeding may come back in the future, so you will have to return to the doctor for frequent checkups and possibly additional laser treatments. Research finds that scatter laser treatment is very effective, potentially preserving good vision for more than a decade.

In selected situations, photocoagulation may be even more

FOCAL LASER TREATMENT　　　　BOX 6-5

Laser burns

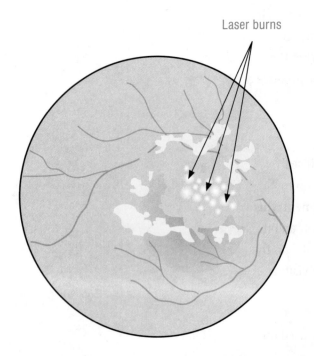

SCATTER LASER TREATMENT　　　　BOX 6-6

Laser burns

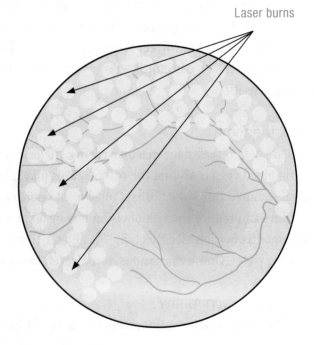

effective when combined with an anti-VEGF drug such as Lucentis or Avastin.

Vitrectomy surgery

If you have a lot of bleeding into the vitreous that has blocked your vision, or you develop scar tissue that leads to a retinal detachment, you may need vitrectomy surgery to remove it. This surgery removes the vitreous gel that has been clouded by blood, and replaces it with saline solution to preserve the correct shape and pressure of the eye. Vitrectomy is performed under local or general anesthesia, and is usually done as outpatient surgery, although it sometimes requires an overnight hospital stay.

The doctor will perform the surgery with tiny instruments guided by looking through a microscope suspended over your eye. After inserting a delicate light probe, the doctor will use a special cutter to slice and extract the vitreous gel. A small tube pumps saline solution in to replace the vitreous gel that is removed. The doctor may also remove scar tissue if it is pulling the retina away from the wall of the eye. This allows a detached retina to settle back into place. The doctor may place a temporary gas bubble in the eye to get the retina to settle into place.

After vitrectomy surgery

After the surgery your eye may be red, swollen and sensitive to light. You will need to wear an eye patch for a while and use antibiotic drops to prevent infection. You may need to position your head in a particular way if the doctor places a gas bubble in the eye, to help your retina reattach. There is a slight risk of complications, including recurring bleeding or glaucoma.

It may take several weeks for your vision to clear fully, but if you have lost sight due to bleeding into the vitreous, the procedure can restore your vision. However, if you have lost sight because of a retinal detachment that involves the center of your retina, the macula, you may still have significant vision loss, even after a successful surgery.

Remain vigilant post-surgery

It is important to note that scatter laser treatment and vitrectomy reduce the risk of blindness to less than five percent when done early enough, but the treatments do not cure proliferative retinopathy. You will always be at risk for new bleeding that can threaten your sight, especially if your diabetes is not well controlled. You will have to be alert for signs of recurring problems and you may need to be treated again.

Under development

There is some hope of improved treatments for diabetic retinopathy in the future. Researchers are studying new therapies that may prevent abnormal blood vessels from forming in the first place, or that treat existing abnormal blood vessels.

Other new treatments under investigation are the topical eye drop mecamylamine and steroid injections.

7 COPING WITH COMPROMISED VISION

BOX 7-1

If you are one of the 25 million blind or visually impaired Americans, you should know that the loss of vision doesn't have to mean the loss of your independence.

Vision rehabilitation services

There are many adaptive devices and coping strategies that can enable you to live a full and independent life. Unfortunately, less than 10 percent of older people with vision impairment take advantage of vision rehabilitation services. This may be due to lack of knowledge about the help that's available, or a lack of money, since many services are not covered by insurance.

Too often, older people do not seek help because they accept impaired vision as a normal part of aging. This is a myth. Healthy eyes do not lose their ability to see as you age; rather, impaired vision is a sign of eye disease that may be treatable. So if you're having trouble recognizing faces, reading, sewing or working under normal lighting conditions, a number of specialists can work together to improve your vision, and help you cope with vision loss (see Box 7-1, "Your team of vision specialists").

Low-vision specialist

A low-vision specialist can evaluate your current vision, and prescribe any necessary adaptive devices or therapies. Medicare usually covers these evaluations, though coverage varies from state to state. Medicare now covers at least some low-vision rehabilitation services as well. Private insurance may cover low-vision evaluations and visual aids, but you should check with your carrier.

Low-vision aids

Most people with low vision retain some usable vision that can be retrained to cope with daily tasks. Adaptive devices, such as high-powered magnifiers or closed-circuit television can help you read, watch TV and do many of the other activities you enjoy. Similarly, certain digital tablet computers have proven to be remarkably effective reading aids, boosting both reading speed and comfort, and smartphones and e-book readers can compensate for visual

Your team of vision specialists

Using a team approach is the best way to deal with vision loss. Consult these specialists if you're having difficulty with your vision:

- **Ophthalmologist:** A medical doctor (M.D.) who is trained to diagnose vision problems and provide medical and surgical care for all eye conditions.

- **Optometrist:** A professional (O.D.) who is licensed by the state to provide eye exams, glasses and contact lenses. In some states, optometrists can prescribe drugs for certain eye conditions.

- **Low-vision specialist:** A specialist who can prescribe magnifiers, telescopes and other optical aids.

- **Occupational therapist:** A therapist who can teach you how to use optical aids, and how to get around more easily with low vision.

- **Physical therapist:** A therapist who can help you improve your balance and show you how to use a cane or walker if you need one.

- **Social worker or psychologist:** A therapist who can help you cope with the emotional repercussions of low vision.

- **Local elder care organization:** To find out about driver rehabilitation and other services in your area call 1-800-677-1116 or visit www.eldercare.gov.

impairments with enlargeable fonts, voice features, and other convenient attributes, according to a study presented at the 2012 annual meeting of the Association for Research in Vision and Ophthalmology. A number of special devices are available—and there's probably something to assist you with just about any work task or hobby you'd like to pursue. You may need to be trained to use them safely and effectively. Here's a quick look at the major categories of low-vision aids:

Digital devices such as smartphones and tablet computers

These enable enlarged font sizes, brighter screens, and GPS and voice features to navigate more easily. Superior backlit screens, for example, on the iPad™, increase reading speed and comfort, (see Box 7-2, "Tablets boost speed and comfort for readers with moderate loss of central vision").

Magnifying glasses

These can be handheld, placed in a stand or fitted into your glasses to help you see small objects more clearly and read more easily.

NEW FINDING   BOX 7-2

Tablets boost speed and comfort for readers with moderate loss of central vision

Certain digital tablet computers can be surprisingly effective reading aids for those with moderate loss of central vision, as from macular degeneration, or diabetic retinopathy, according to a study presented at the 2012 annual meeting of the American Academy of Ophthalmology. Use of tablets boosted reading speed by an average of 15 words per minute.

However, some tablets were more effective than others. Using an iPad™ set on 18 point font, all 100 study subjects gained *at least* 42 words per minute, as compared to reading print, while Kindle readers gained an *average* of only 12 words per minute. The digital instruments were most helpful to those with the poorest vision.

The key to the iPad's superior benefit is the back-lit screen, which makes reading easier regardless of each patient's level of visual acuity. That screen helps with contrast, that is, the patients' ability see objects—letters, in this case—as distinct from the background. The original Kindle, used in this study, lacks a back-lit screen.

The research was conducted at the Robert Wood Johnson Medical School in New Jersey.

Telescopes

These might be fitted onto your glasses to help you watch a movie or a play.

Closed-circuit television

These devices enlarge the lettering in books or magazines and display them on a monitor. Handheld versions can help you read labels when you're shopping at the supermarket.

Auditory devices

These range from talking thermometers to tools that can read a book out loud. They use electronic speech technology to read the written information.

Filters

These devices can reduce glare and improve contrast, making it easier to read.

Large-print products

Books, magazines, newspapers, computer software and clocks are all available in large-print formats for the vision impaired. Some devices have a 'talking' feature that reads the words aloud.

Rehabilitation therapy

You also may need certain forms of rehabilitation therapy. A mobility specialist can teach you how to get around with your existing vision by using a cane or a seeing-eye dog. A therapist may evaluate your home and help you improve the lighting, or add colorful labels or tactile markings to everyday objects so you can find them. Or the therapist may teach you new ways to cook, clean and do other household tasks to keep you independent.

Safety changes in your home

You may need to make some changes in your home to prevent falls. Studies have shown that people with low vision, particularly those with impaired depth perception, are at an increased risk of injuries from falls. Here are some simple things you can do to prevent this problem:

‣ Use non-slip mats in tubs and showers.
‣ Remove area rugs and other hazards, such as books, papers or other clutter, that might cause tripping or falls.
‣ Install more lighting throughout your home, particularly on stairs.

- Arrange furniture so you have a clear path to walk through each room.
- Use the right glasses for the occasion. One study found that switching from multifocal to single-vision glasses while outdoors could reduce the risk of falls by 40 percent. However, the change in eyewear did slightly increase the risk of falls and non-fall-related injuries in older adults who didn't get outside often, which is why it's important for eye doctors to assess their patients' activity levels before prescribing glasses.

Counseling for depression

Many people have trouble adjusting to vision loss; it can be one of the most debilitating disabilities. Depression is common in patients with low vision. If you are feeling depressed about your vision problems, ask your low-vision specialist to refer you to a counselor. You can also join a support group for the visually impaired and their families.

There's increasing evidence that low-vision services improve patients' abilities to perform specific tasks and remain active. These services also help improve quality of life, reduce depression and improve coping skills. Research finds that seniors who take part in a weekly low-vision rehabilitation program have great improvements in vision, reading ability, information processing and their ability to get around.

8 CONCLUSION

We hope this report has given you a better understanding of the four most common age-related eye diseases. These conditions have visually impaired millions of older Americans, and those numbers could skyrocket as Baby Boomers age. The statistics are particularly tragic, given that about half of all people who become blind could save their sight with vigilant screening and early treatment.

Innovative research underway

Research into diseases of the eyes and vision loss is moving forward at a rapid pace. Scientists are innovating in myriad ways that promise to mitigate and prevent some eye conditions. Emerging technologies, including stem cells, synthetic corneas, and retinal implants, offer the hope that some blind people will see again.

Despite aging, and the rising risk of impaired vision that entails, you can take precautions that will boost your chances of preserving your sight. We hope that after reading this special report, you'll make an appointment to see your ophthalmologist for your annual eye exam, if you haven't had one already. **Regular vision screening** is the single most important thing you can do to protect and preserve your sight. The next step is to make **simple lifestyle changes** that may help prevent vision loss, such as losing weight and stopping smoking. Finally, be vigilant about any vision problems that do arise, and act quickly to have them treated.

APPENDIX I: GLOSSARY

Age-Related Macular Degeneration: A group of conditions that cause deterioration of the macula and can lead to the loss of central vision. There are two forms of age-related macular degeneration: dry and wet.

Anterior Chamber: The space between the cornea and the lens in the front of the eye.

Antioxidant: A chemical that protects cells from damage that can occur from light, stress or normal metabolic processes. Antioxidants such as vitamins E and C are often found in foods.

Aqueous: The clear fluid produced by the ciliary body that fills the anterior chamber of the eye and gives the front of the eye its shape. Too much aqueous can cause eye pressure to rise, leading to glaucoma.

Cataract: Clouding of the lens that prevents a clear image from forming on the retina, blurring vision.

Choroid: A middle layer of the eye, sandwiched between the retina and the sclera. It is made up of blood vessels that bring nutrition to the retina and other structures, and helps remove wastes.

Ciliary Body: A ring of tissue that produces the aqueous and helps change the shape of the lens as needed.

Cones: Light-sensitive, cone-shaped cells in the retina, particularly in the macula, that help us see detail, shape and color. They function best in daylight.

Cornea: The clear membrane in front of the eye that helps focus light so we can see.

Diabetic Retinopathy: A wide range of changes to the retina that are caused by diabetes and can compromise vision.

Drusen: A yellow deposit found under the macula that is typically related to dry age-related macular degeneration. It is thought to be an accumulation of waste products.

Floaters: Particles that float in the vitreous and cast shadows on the retina. They appear as spots that interfere with vision.

Fovea: The tiny center of the macula. It carries a high concentration of the cone cells that help us see colors.

Free Radical: A molecule that causes damage to a cell or tissue.

Glaucoma: A condition that occurs when increased eye pressure damages the optic nerve. It can lead to vision loss.

Iris: The colored part of the eye, responsible for controlling how much light enters the eye through the pupil.

Laser: An acronym for Light Amplification by Stimulated Emission of Radiation. A high-energy light source that is used to cut, burn or dissolve tissue in many eye procedures.

Legal Blindness: A condition in which a person cannot see better than 20/200 in his or her best eye, even with glasses or contact lenses.

Lens: A thin, clear structure that focuses light on the retina to produce an image.

Low Vision: Impaired vision that cannot be corrected and interferes with the ability to perform everyday activities.

Macula: The small part of the retina responsible for the most finely detailed central vision.

Optic Nerve: A bundle of nerve fibers that carries an image from the retina to the brain, where it is processed.

Pupil: The black center of the iris, which changes size to reduce or increase the amount of light that enters the eye.

Retina: The lining of the back of the eye. It is full of light-sensitive cells and nerves that pick up the image focused on the retina by the cornea and lens and send it to the optic nerve.

Rods: Light-sensitive cells in the retina that help you see in dark conditions.

Sclera: The white of the eye.

Vitreous: The gel that gives the eye its shape. It fills the area between the lens and the retina.

APPENDIX II: RESOURCES

American Academy of Ophthalmology
P.O. Box 7424
San Francisco, CA 94120-7424
415-561-8500
www.aao.org

American Council of the Blind
2200 Wilson Boulevard, Suite 650
Arlington, VA 22201
800-424-8666
www.acb.org

American Foundation for the Blind
2 Penn Plaza, Suite 1102
New York, NY 10121
800-232-5463
www.afb.org

Lighthouse International
111 E. 59th Street
New York, NY 10022-1202
800-829-0500
www.lighthouse.org

National Eye Institute
Information Office
31 Center Drive MSC 2510
Bethesda, MD 20892-2510
301-496-5248
www.nei.nih.gov

Eye Health Organizations Database:
http://www.nei.nih.gov/health/resourceSearch.asp

National Federation of the Blind
200 East Wells Street
Baltimore, MD 21230
410-659-9314
www.nfb.org

Prevent Blindness America
211 West Wacker Drive
Suite 1700
Chicago, Il 60606
800-331-2020
www.preventblindness.org

APPENDIX III: FINANCIAL RESOURCES

If you've been avoiding routine eye exams because of the costs involved, be aware that you may be eligible for assistance. People with diabetes, a high risk of glaucoma or who are over 65 may qualify for free eye care through EyeCare America. This service of the American Academy of Ophthalmology will refer you to an ophthalmologist in your area, and provide you with an exam at no out-of-pocket cost to you (though your insurance may be billed). For more information call 1-800-222-EYES, or visit www.eyecareamerica.org. People with low incomes and no vision insurance may be eligible for eye care through Vision USA, a program of the American Optometric Association. For more information call 1-800-766-4466, or visit www.optometryscharity.org/vision-usa/. Importantly, Medicare has recently added an annual glaucoma screening benefit so once you reach Medicare age, be sure to take advantage of this (www.medicare.gov).